THE PSYCHOLOGY OF PRENATAL DEVELOPMENT

This important book introduces the basics of prenatal psychology and works through the current scientific findings in the psychology and psychosomatics of pregnancy and birth. Through exploring bio-psycho-social relationships, as well as historical and cultural perspectives, this interdisciplinary approach easily breaks down specialist discussions into easy-to-understand concepts.

Bridging the gap between foetal programming and psychological research and practice, this accessible book presents the history of the field and the basic concepts of prenatal development before exploring the behavioural dimensions of life before, during and immediately after birth. Topics include sensory and emotional development in the womb, perception and brain development, the influence of environmental factors and prenatal imprinting and long-term effects. The author also delves into the concept of attachment and support and analyses body symptoms, sensations, feelings and inner images in dreams and imaginations, through the role of art creations and biographical narratives. As a whole, this book provides a therapeutic synopsis of the entire existence, which begins with conception.

Explaining how experiences in the prenatal period influence basic psychological imprints across the lifespan, this book is an essential resource for students in a wide range of interrelated disciplines, including developmental psychology, paediatric medicine, neuroscience, infancy and early child development, nursing, social work and early childhood education. It may also be of interest to researchers, clinicians and related professionals.

Klaus Evertz works as psycho-, art- and body therapist in his own practice as well as at the Dr. Mildred-Scheel-Academy, University Hospital Cologne, Germany, and until 2021, at the Center for Palliative Medicine, University Hospital Cologne. A painter and cultural psychologist, his research is in images as forms of consciousness, and he teaches at the Universities of Cologne and Dresden, the Nürtingen University of Art Therapy and the Nürtingen-Geislingen University of Economics, Germany.

"After hundreds of years of research into the reality of prenatal and birth life, it is now possible to provide this comprehensive overview of Prenatal Psychology. The reader can prepare for an adventure of expanding inner perception and knowledge".

Dr. med. Ludwig Janus, *Facharzt für Psychotherapeutische Medizin, Pränatalpsychologe und Psychohistoriker, Institut für Pränatale Psychologie und Medizin, Germany*

"Klaus Evertz's new book brings intelligent, scientifically supported, evidence-based, peer reviewed studies into the realm of vanguard mainstream psychology, within everyone's grasp. Though he is writing from the frontier, his words convey what is self-evident to earnest ordinary human beings, words entwined with the disciplined rigor we expect from our pioneers. What a pleasure to recognize, as you are reading, that this makes absolute sense. As if he is putting language to something you have intuitively already known".

Karlton Terry, *Pre and Perinatal Workshop Leader, New Mexico, USA*

THE PSYCHOLOGY OF PRENATAL DEVELOPMENT

A Therapeutic Synopsis
of Human Existence

Klaus Evertz

With the collaboration of Nadja Evertz and Ludwig Janus

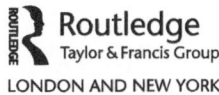

Routledge
Taylor & Francis Group

LONDON AND NEW YORK

Cover image: *Colouraction* by Klaus Evertz
Farbhandlung 8.2.23. 50x50x0,3 cm, oil on HDF

First published 2025
by Routledge
4 Park Square, Milton Park, Abingdon, Oxon OX14 4RN

and by Routledge
605 Third Avenue, New York, NY 10158

Routledge is an imprint of the Taylor & Francis Group, an informa business

British Library Cataloguing-in-Publication Data
A catalogue record for this book is available from the British Library

ISBN: 978-1-032-76848-9 (hbk)
ISBN: 978-1-032-76136-7 (pbk)
ISBN: 978-1-003-48024-2 (ebk)

DOI: 10.4324/9781003480242

Typeset in Optima
by codeMantra

Please visit the author's website at www.klausevertz.de

CONTENTS

1

INTRODUCTION

Preliminary remark

This book attempts to summarise the most important aspects of prenatal human development from a psychological perspective. As it deals with bio-psycho-social relationships and historical and cultural aspects, it is an interdisciplinary and transdisciplinary book. It requires the reader to repeatedly step back from the individual specialist discussions and attempt to summarise them on a meta-level. This always involves self-awareness and self-reflection, as prenatal psychology, like all other scientific topics, can ultimately only be evaluated and understood from a subjective perspective when objective information is taken in. However, the guiding principle of this book is psychology and human science-based psychotherapeutic experience with babies, children, adolescents, adults and dying people.

Some of the information and stories may be particularly moving for the reader. If you, as a reader, notice that particular feelings of happiness and joy, but also of sadness and grief, of pain arise or you simply have the feeling that an irritating effect is occurring, it is worth pausing and asking yourself the question: what does what I have just read perhaps have to do with my own life? What memories are being touched upon that were perhaps previously unconscious? What thoughts about my own family system, my own development, my pregnancy and birth are stimulated by the reading?

Many people only come to these deeper perspectives on their own lives in times of crisis. That is why this book could only have been written from the 'narratives' of thousands of pregnant couples and patients, from babies to the dying, who showed and depicted themselves through body symptoms, sensations, feelings, inner images in dreams and imaginations, art creations,

DOI: 10.4324/9781003480242-1

behavioural patterns and biographical narratives. But it was always about attempts at a therapeutic synopsis of the entire existence, which begins with conception. In therapeutic contexts, the laws of human existence are more clearly reflected than in everyday life, which is why medical and psychotherapeutic phenomenology is indispensable in the study of the human psyche.

It is a particular challenge to establish a real inner relationship to the experiences of pre-linguistic times.

> "Strong in the egg", Pharaoh Ramses II on his prenatal period
> "…Nescire autem quid ante quam natus sis acciderit, id est semper esse puerum".
> Marcus Tullius Cicero, Orator 120
> "If we do not gain access to our existence before birth, we always remain a child".

The theory of prenatal psychology establishes an expanded nosology. Psychological and somatic illnesses in childhood, adolescence and adulthood can be increasingly clearly attributed to epigenetics and the psychological circumstances of pregnancy.

At the same time, this theory is the basis for a bio-psycho-social medicine of the future and thus also a new theoretical foundation for comprehensive psychosomatics, in which biological genetics and transgenerational family-systemic psychology/psychotherapy complement each other just as much as the epigenetics of pregnancy and prenatal psychology. The realisation and progress of prenatal-based psychotherapy is the ability to differentiate precisely between transgenerational, prenatal and postnatal trauma (Evertz 2020, 2022).

This book introduces the basics of prenatal psychology and deals with the current scientific findings in the psychology and psychosomatics of pregnancy and birth. It builds a bridge between the biological-medical research of foetal programming and psychological and psychotherapeutic research and practice.

Prenatal psychology is particularly concerned with research on two levels:

1 The psychological level of the generative transmission of bio-psycho-social information during conception and pregnancy to the child,
2 Research into the potential experiential realities of the child in the prenatal phase of life from the first cell onwards,
3 The conditions of conscious parenthood as the strongest resilience factor.

This raises epistemological, scientific-theoretical and also psychohistorical, psychotherapeutic and biopsychological questions, which we outline in this book.

The biographical space of the prenatal period and birth has received increasing attention in recent years in terms of its significance for medicine and psychotherapy. Formative experiences for the later attitude to life and sense of self are made in the prenatal period, while the birth experience influences our later handling of changes and our own individuation possibilities. The significance of these experiences has been analysed on a qualitative level in various psychotherapeutic settings. These observations are now supported by empirical research: prenatal stress influences later behaviour in the sense of greater sensitivity to stress, and the prenatal atmosphere shapes the synaptic connections of the developing brain and thus dispositions towards certain behaviours, emotional attitudes and moods. And "foetal programming" is used to fine-tune the physiological control of the organism. Physical and psychological dispositions to illness and the aetiology of postnatal illnesses become clearer, thus enabling extended therapeutic concepts. These empirical findings correspond to observations from various psychotherapeutic settings. At the same time, the prenatal period contains the vital primal experiences of one's own vitality and strength, which can become inaccessible due to traumatic stress and which need to be reconnected to in happy therapy.

Introduction: love

Therapeutic culture in the 20th and 21st centuries is a civilisational development in the tradition of the Enlightenment. Kant's dictum of liberation from self-imposed immaturity through reason is still relevant and forward-looking. Humanity is far from having reached the end of the road as long as sustainable destructions such as environmental degradation, wars, religious fundamentalism, extremist political movements and global economic injustices continue to sabotage and jeopardise coexistence and a peaceful global society. Modernity is still an unfinished project (Habermas). Psychology as the science of the conditions of human behaviour, human bonding and relationship skills, human feelings, emotions and thinking is, as part of the human and natural sciences, the interface between practical philosophy as theory and therapeutic practice.

Prenatal psychology examines the beginning of human life. In a different form than biology, anthropology, archaeology, evolutionary theory of knowledge, etc., it examines the phenomenon of life at its ontogenetic origin.

The only real transcendence is children. Could it be that we have so far paid too little attention to the fact that the phenomenon of passing on life, which repeats itself with every generation, is not just a biochemical and sexual process but an extremely complex and sensitive bio-psycho-social process that involves so many imprints that much is already decided there that most people in adult life consider to be coincidental or only understand in terms of fate?

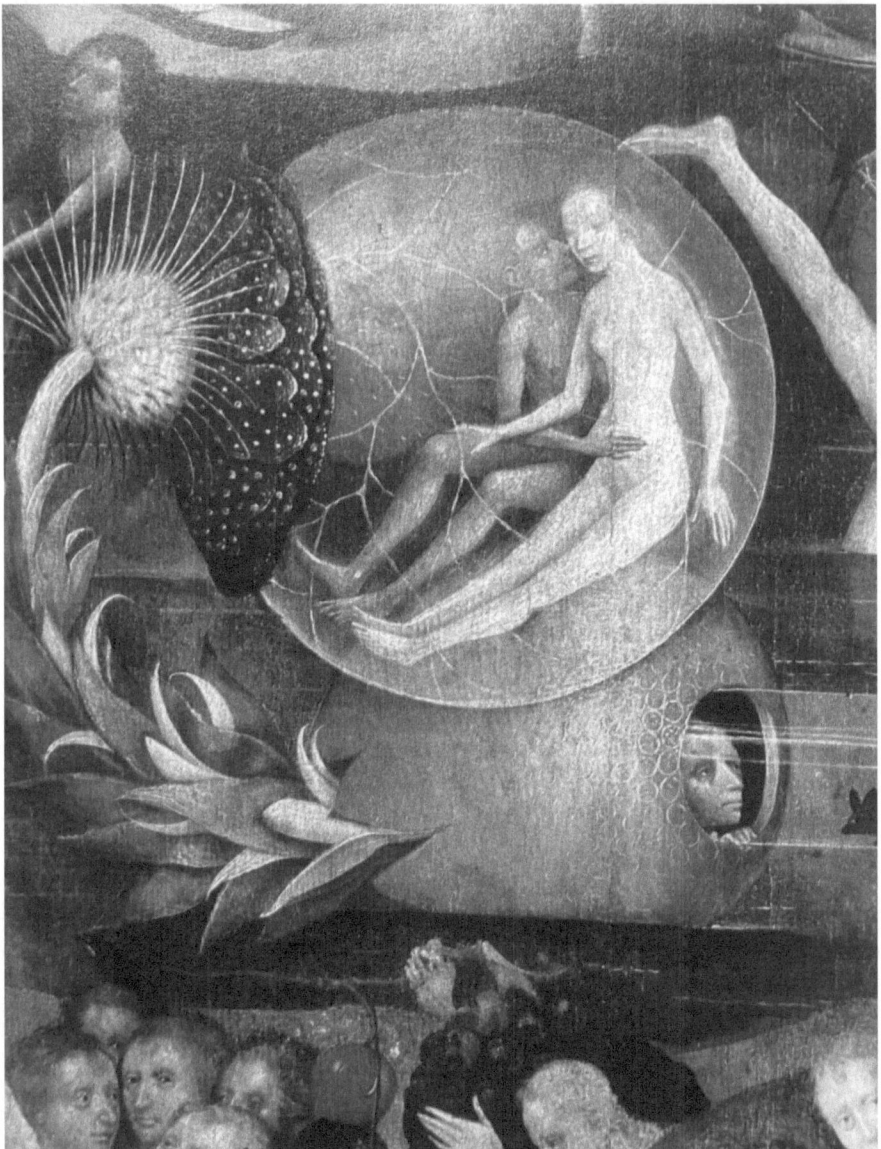

FIGURE 1.1 Man and woman: The origin of all human life.

Prenatal psychology is a research and scientific discipline that has developed within psychology over the last 50 years. It examines the emotional conditions of conception, pregnancy and birth in all their bonding and relationship qualities and investigates the connection between prenatal imprinting and postnatal effects on the entire human lifespan.

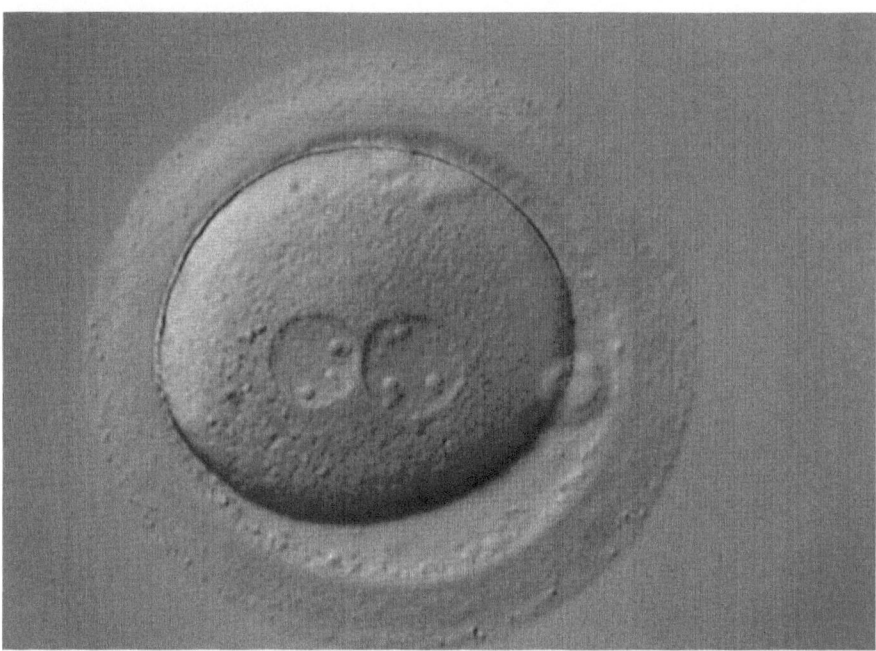

FIGURE 1.2 Detail from the *Garden of Earthly Delights* by Hieronymus Bosch (1490/1500) and modern photo of a zygote, the union of paternal and maternal genetic material.

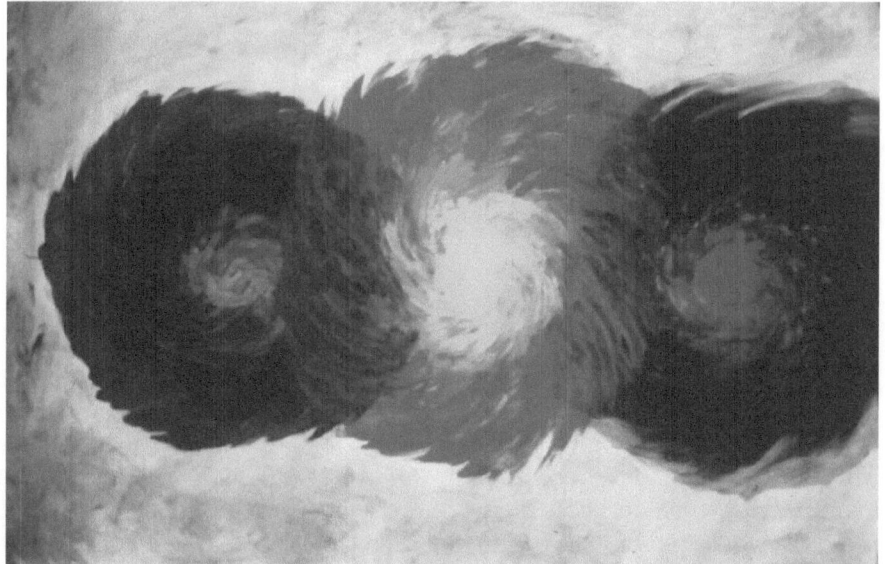

FIGURE 1.3 The first triangulation, painting of a client's conception.

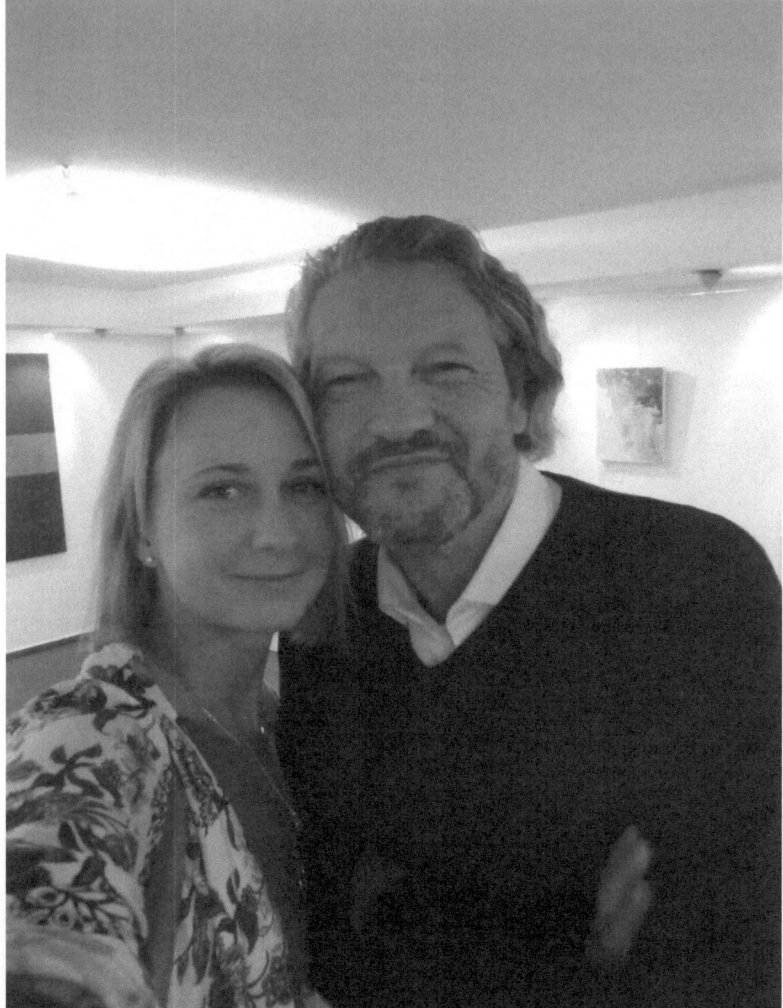

FIGURE 1.4 A modern couple.

Two become three.

The core of every psychotherapy is ultimately the patient's questions: Can I love? And: Am I loved? Where do I feel safe?

The greatest real longing of all people is for great love. For a trusting, peaceful, pleasurable, varied and, if possible, lifelong relationship. All studies in all cultures reveal this core theme of every life. People want to love and be loved. They want to be recognised and seen. They want to feel accepted for who they are and experience warmth, tenderness and exchange in a secure bond. This deep longing and also its disappointment is the main theme at all cultural levels and in all art forms, with the themes of transience, violence, pain and death. The context is always that destructive aggression and agonising forms of love are always the result of disappointed expectations of love.

Where does the longing for love actually come from?

"The invention of the mother" (Slotderdijk) in evolution happened in the transition to mammals, which differed from their predecessors and began to let the offspring mature in the body of the female animals, i.e. intracorporeally instead of extra-corporeally, until a certain stage was reached that the child could also survive outside the mother, even if it still needed the care and protection of the parents. The "invention of the mother" was therefore also the invention of the uterus and the placenta and also the invention of a much larger social space and the invention of personal love.

In humans, it takes nine months for the child to grow inside the mother before it can be born. Anthropologists speak of a physiological premature birth of the human being, as it is actually born too early due to the upright gait of the human being. The human child should actually be in the womb for a few more months in order to be more stable and independent. However, the woman's pelvis would then be far too narrow to allow the baby's head to pass through. In contrast to most other mammals, the human child is therefore born very helpless.

What initially appears to be an evolutionary flaw, however, has brought a decisive evolutionary advantage for humans: in order for a human child to survive outside the womb at all, it needs intensive care and nurturing for at least 3 to 5 years, i.e. much longer than most other animal species; otherwise, it dies. This social space of closeness and intimacy, of dependence and special care is an extension of intrauterine existence. Here, humans have learned that altruistic behaviours, caring for another living being and feelings for one's own child, open up an exhausting but also wonderful space of love and recognition, which has ultimately led to the cultural achievements of mankind.

Humans, in their sensitivity and vulnerability, have thus become social beings precisely because of this supposed weakness. They can cope with the dangers of the world with a much greater sociality and creativity beyond their instinctive framework and invent completely new things where all other animal species remain within their instinctive framework.

Neoteny describes the strategy of evolution to bring ever more sensitive and delicate creatures into the world, which are "forced" to develop new life forms precisely because of the greater chance of injury. The mutual reinforcement of external conditions, brain growth and flexibility led to *Homo sapiens*, which is currently the dominant living being in the world.

Human love is therefore actually a deepening and refinement of the sexual instinct, where it is no longer just about reproduction but also about increasing social and empathic qualities of responsibility in bonds and relationships. Humans are therefore still and continue to practise how a human society can be learnt without destructive destruction and violence.

The concept of love exists in 147 of the 166 cultures analysed. Depending on the study, a stable couple relationship is one of the most important goals in life for 80 or even 99 per cent of those surveyed. This can be easily explained by evolutionary biology: In a stable love relationship, the man could be sure that he was raising his children and not someone else's; and the woman could assume that he was providing the 100,000 extra calories she needed during the long breastfeeding period.

(Wellershoff 2024)

The origin of love and the capacity for peaceful human relationships therefore lie in how these can also be learnt and improved. People learn a great deal about these possibilities in the prenatal nine months and the postnatal nine months. A contented and happy mother can give her child much more strength, confidence and the ability to love for life than a fearful or depressed mother. Well-bonded children do not make wars.

Basic concepts of prenatal psychology

1 Transgenerational conditions – preconceptual psychology – systemic psychology: This concept encompasses the genetic and familial factors of the father's and mother's family systems, all of which have an influence on the new child.
2 Periconceptional conditions – periconceptional psychology – systemic psychology: This concept describes the biological and emotional qualities of a couple's unconscious or conscious decision to conceive a child.
3 Prenatal development: This concept refers to the development of the embryo and foetus in the womb. It encompasses the different stages of pregnancy and the associated changes in the foetus' body and brain.
4 Prenatal perception: This concept refers to the foetus' ability to perceive various stimuli from its environment. This includes sounds, movements, touch and even taste senses.
5 Prenatal bonding: This concept refers to the emotional bond between the expectant mother and the unborn child. We now know that this bond develops before and during pregnancy and has an influence on the later parent-child relationship. This also includes the forms of non-relationship, denial, rejection of the child and pregnancy. However, it also includes the quality of the couple's bond and the father's bond with the child. The father's attitude towards the mother and the expectant child also has an effect on the course of the pregnancy and the quality of the birth.
6 Prenatal learning: This concept refers to the foetus's ability to learn and store information from its environment. Studies have shown that babies can recognise certain sounds or voices while still in the womb.

7 Prenatal stress effects: This concept refers to the impact of stress during pregnancy on the unborn child. Research has shown that high levels of stress in the mother and family system can have negative effects on foetal development.

8 Prenatal environmental factors: This concept refers to the various environmental factors to which the foetus is exposed during pregnancy. These include nutrition, smoking, alcohol consumption and environmental toxins, all of which can have an impact on foetal development.

9 Prenatal stimulation: This concept refers to the targeted stimulation of the foetus during pregnancy. This includes, for example, music or gentle touch, which are intended to promote the development of the foetus.

10 Prenatal diagnostics: This concept refers to the various medical tests and examinations carried out during pregnancy to detect possible genetic or developmental problems in the foetus at an early stage.

11 Prenatal intervention: This concept refers to measures that can be taken to treat or prevent potential problems or developmental delays in the foetus. This includes, for example, medical treatments or therapies.

12 Prenatal bonding support: This concept refers to measures and activities aimed at strengthening the bond between the expectant mother and the unborn child (Figure 1.5). This includes, for example, talking to the baby in the womb or singing songs and all levels of conscious and unconscious awareness of this new relationship with a new human being. The more intuitively and consciously the father and mother feel and accept their new role, the more the child can feel itself (Evertz et al. 2021).

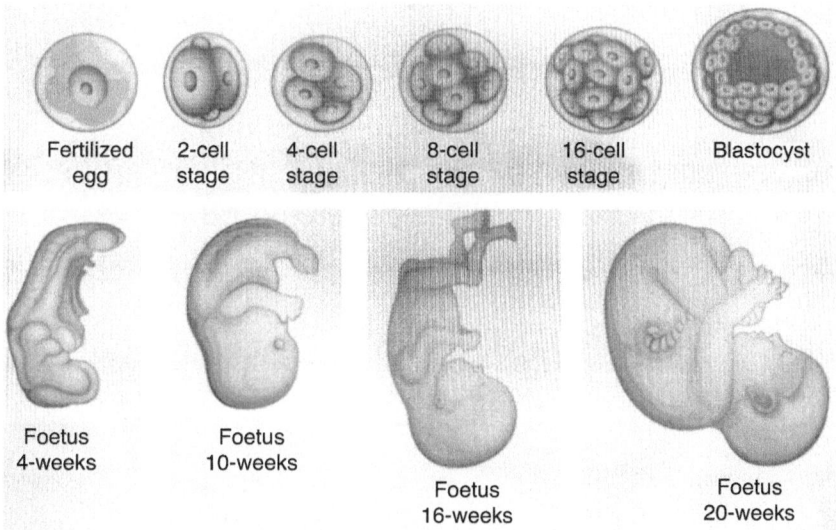

| Fertilized egg | 2-cell stage | 4-cell stage | 8-cell stage | 16-cell stage | Blastocyst |

Foetus 4-weeks

Foetus 10-weeks

Foetus 16-weeks

Foetus 20-weeks

FIGURE 1.5 Models of physical development up to 20 weeks (Shutterstock).

Literature

Evertz K (2020) "Das innere Kind oder das "innere Kind"? – Transgenerationale und pränatale Traumaschichten". *Forum für Kunsttherapien, Zeitschrift des Fachverbandes für Gestaltende Psychotherapie und Kunsttherapie GPK*. Aarburg, Schweiz, 30–36.

Evertz K (2022) "Die Welt neu spüren – Die transgenerational-systemisch und pränatal fundierte methodenintegrative Psychotherapie – Integrative Kunst- und Körpertherapie". In: Klippel-Heidekrüger M, Janus L (eds.) *Vielfältige Zugänge zum vorsprachlichen und geburtlichen Erleben*. Mattes Verlag, Heidelberg, 271–292.

Evertz K, Janus L, Linder R (2021) *Handbook of prenatal and perinatal psychology - Integrating research and practice*. Springer Nature, Heidelberg, New York.

Wellershoff M (2024) "Warum manche Paare für immer zusammenbleiben – und viele andere nicht". In: *Spiegel*, 11.1.24.– https://www.spiegel.de/partnerschaft/langzeitbeziehungen-warum-manche-paare-fuer-immer-zusammenbleiben-und-andere-nicht-a-53d3a0b2-088c-4bc6-9927-b2da2dc7f8cc

2

HISTORICAL DEVELOPMENT OF PRENATAL PSYCHOLOGY

This chapter provides a brief overview of the history of prenatal psychology and the fundamental importance of this new discipline. Prenatal psychology developed on the basis of depth psychological observations that allowed conclusions to be drawn about prenatal trauma, stress or other formative situations. Today, prenatal psychology is a specialised discipline that investigates both the generative transmission of bio-psycho-social information during pregnancy and the realities of experience in the prenatal phase of life. The findings of the natural sciences are just as integrated as those of the humanities and cultural sciences.

Sandor Ferenczi published *Developmental Stages of the Sense of Reality* in 1913 and *An Attempt at a Genital Theory* in 1924, thereby laying an important foundation for psychoanalytical considerations on the beginning of psychic life. Freud was also aware of the intrauterine dimension but did not develop it theoretically (Janus 2000).

Ferenczi writes in the *Developmental Stages of the Sense of Reality* about the connection between feelings of omnipotence and the initial intrauterine basic feelings:

> In this state, the human being lives like a parasite of the womb... so if the human being has a soul life in the womb, even if unconscious – and it would be nonsensical to believe that the soul only begins to work at the moment of birth – he must get the impression from his existence that he is actually omnipotent. But the embryo could claim this of itself, because it always has everything it needs to satisfy its instincts, which is why it has nothing to desire, it has no needs. The child's delusion of grandeur and its own omnipotence is therefore at least not an empty delusion. The child and

DOI: 10.4324/9781003480242-2

the obsessive-compulsive neurotic do not demand anything impossible from reality if they cannot be dissuaded from the fact that their wishes must be fulfilled. They only demand the return of a state that once existed, the "good old days" when they were omnipotent (period of unconditional omnipotence)... But if you observe the other behaviour of the newborn child, you get the impression that it is not at all pleased by the rude disturbance of the undesirable peace it enjoyed in the womb, indeed that it longs to return to this situation. The carers instinctively recognise this desire in the child, and as soon as it expresses its displeasure by fidgeting and crying, they deliberately place it in a position that is as similar as possible to the situation in the womb...or they reproduce the quiet and rhythmic monotonous stimuli that the child was not spared even in utero, the rocking movements when the mother walks, the mother's heartbeat, the muffled sound that penetrates from outside into the body by rocking the child and humming monotonous, rhythmic lullabies to it. I convinced myself that every later sleep is nothing other than a periodically repeating regression to the stage of magical-hallucinatory omnipotence and with its help to the absolute omnipotence of the womb situation....

(Ferenczi 1913, p. 62ff)

Ferenczi's relatively early death prevented him from writing a later work in which he could have developed the foundations for prenatal psychology. At the same time, Otto Rank, Freud's student and secretary, continued to work on these ideas and published the book *The Trauma of Birth* in 1924, in which he theorised his experiences from the analyses in which the patients tended towards birth fantasies and rebirth symbolism towards the end of the therapy. The determination of the end of the therapy thus provoked birth fantasies:

In a series of analyses that were usually successfully completed, I noticed that in the final phase of the analysis, the healing process was regularly depicted by the unconscious in the typical birth symbolism that we are largely already familiar with.... I had noticed that this was obviously the familiar fantasy of rebirth in which the patient's will to recover clothed his healing....until one day, in a particularly clear case, I realised that the strongest resistance to the resolution of the transference libido in the final phase of the analysis was expressed in the form of the earliest infantile fixations to the mother, that this fixation to the mother, which seemed to underlie the analytic fixation, contained the earliest, purely physiological relationship to the maternal body. This also made the regularity of the rebirth fantasy understandable and its real substrate analytically comprehensible. The patient's "rebirth fantasy" proved to be simply a repetition of his birth in the analysis, whereby the detachment from the analyst's libido object seemed to correspond to an exact reproduction of the first detachment from the first libido object, the newborn from the mother... The analysis thus ultimately proves to be a subsequent resolution of the imperfectly overcome birth trauma...From this it follows that the actual transference libido which we have to resolve analytically in both sexes is the maternal one, as it was given in the prenatal, physiological bond between mother and child...

(Rank 1924, p. 5ff)

Since the publication of Otto Rank's book *The Trauma of Birth* in 1924, there have been increasing observations in psychoanalytic and psychotherapeutic treatments that patients with a wide range of disorders and illnesses have made conscious and unconscious aetiological references to their first years of life and also to their pregnancy and birth. In stories about their origins, their family of origin and their early childhood, connections emerged that explained the current illness and life crisis. In many cases, these subjective aetiologies could also be objectively verified and recognised, particularly because the psychotherapeutic treatment was also noticeably successful and sustainable when the therapist took these subjective aetiologies seriously and took them into account in the treatment.

However, these therapeutic observations and findings met with increasing resistance from Freud himself and the emerging field of psychoanalysis at the time. There were fears that the public, who were already overwhelmed by the findings of psychoanalysis, would turn away completely if the psychological roots of adult life were explored not only in childhood but even in birth and pregnancy.

We must not forget that psychoanalysis emerged in an empire, a completely patriarchal, authority-fixated and hierarchically orientated world in which feelings in general, but especially the feelings of women and children and the maternal dimension of relationships were treated more as decoration and accessory than as an existential reality.

In the ensuing debate between Freud and Rank, Freud continued to speak of "birth fantasies", while Rank spoke of "birth reality". Rank ultimately accused Freud of paying too much attention to the role of the patient's father in the analysis and underestimating the maternal dimension. Freud never really wanted to recognise the "bad mother" (Whitebook 2018; Janus 2023).

Freud and the main tradition of psychoanalysis largely denied the importance of the maternal-feminine dimension and the assumption of a prenatal soul life but at least pushed ahead with research into the infant and toddler period. This research is particularly associated with the names of Anna Freud and Melanie Klein.

Two strands of pre- and perinatal psychology now emerged:

1 Rank had to leave the Psychoanalytical Association but continued his work in Paris and New York, where he became a pioneer of humanistic

psychology and transpersonal psychology, which produced important representatives of prenatal psychology in the USA, namely Arthur Janov and Stanislav Grof and later William Emerson. Frank Lake and Ronald Laing were among the most important pioneers in England.

2 Hans Gustav Graber published *The Ambivalence of the Child* in 1924, in which he dealt with the tension of the child between regression and development and also included a prenatal soul life and the birth process. He was able to develop a niche within psychoanalysis, which led to the founding of the "International Study Group for Prenatal Psychology" (ISPP) in 1971 (Janus 2000, 2014, 2021).

It was not until the Austrian psychoanalyst Otto Rank discovered the traumatic aspects of birth and their continued effects in experience in 1924 (Rank 1924) that the Hungarian-American psychoanalyst Nandor Fodor (Fodor 1949) and others discovered the traumatic aspects and their continued effects in all subsequent experience and behaviour in 1949. Due to the restriction of the psychoanalytic tradition to postnatal development, which corresponded to public awareness at the time, further research into these connections took place within the framework of humanistic psychology, which is associated with the names of Arthur Janov, Stanislav Grof and William Emerson in the USA and Frank Lake and Ronald Laing in England (Janus 2000, 2014, 2021).

In the 1970s and 1980s, specialist scientific societies also developed which, under the name of "prenatal psychology", offered a scientific forum for observing the experiential and behavioural impact of prenatal and birth experiences: in 1971, the "Studiengemeinschaft für Pränatale Psychologie" (Study Society for Prenatal Psychology), still from a psychoanalytical background, which later, from 1986, formed itself in an interdisciplinary and transdisciplinary manner as the "International Society for Prenatal and Perinatal Psychology and Medicine" (ISPPM) (www.isppm.de) and then in 1981 the North American "Association for Prenatal and Perinatal Psychology and Health" (APPPAH) (www.birthpsychology.com). Both societies organised and still organise regular congresses and publish the results of their research in their own journals and publications. There are also two societies for prenatal psychology in Italy (www.anep.it and www.anpep.it). In Heidelberg, Germany, the "Institute for Prenatal Psychology and Medicine" (www.pränatalpsychologie.de) endeavours to impart existing knowledge in the fields of psychotherapy, obstetrics and cultural studies.

The collective psychological dimension in history and in society is being researched by the psychohistorical societies in the USA and Germany (www.psychohistory.com, www.gppp.de).

Within this framework, it was then possible to constructively relate the findings of stress research, brain research, epidemiology, epigenetics and observations in various psychotherapeutic settings, which were obtained on different methodological levels. This also applies to the observations of midwives such as Dorothy Garleigh or Verena Schmidt and obstetricians such as Frédérick Leboyer and Michel Odent on the significance of the child's experience before and during birth and its after-effects in later life (Janus 2021a, 2021b).

The focus was on the after-effects of traumatisation because they are clearly reflected in later experience and behaviour and become conspicuous as disruptive factors. However, the above-mentioned observations also opened up the view that it is true for prenatal experiences and conditions as a whole that the child develops before birth in the medium of its mother's emotionality and feelings. The discovery of implicit and procedural memory in the 1970s and 1980s also made it possible to integrate these observations, which initially seemed strange from the perspective of linguistic memory, into a framework of understanding.

From observations in psychoanalytic practice to the pioneers

Freud offered his patients a very supportive therapeutic situation. The patients were allowed to lie down on a couch and say everything that was on their minds when they were able to talk about their current illness, crisis, pain and fears. It became clear that relief and relaxation, solutions and healing of symptoms occurred when their roots could be identified in the biography. This enabled the integration of the patient's feelings, which resulted in a stronger and more resilient identity.

> We found... to our great surprise that the individual hysterical symptoms disappeared immediately and without recurrence when we succeeded in awakening to full brightness the memory of the process which had caused them, and thus also in awakening the accompanying affect, and when the patient then described the process in as much detail as possible and gave words to the affect. Recollection without affect is almost always completely ineffective; the psychic process which originally took place must be repeated as vividly as possible, brought into statum nascendi and then "spoken out"....
>
> *(S. Freud: Studies on Hysteria, p. 85)*

> I only learnt to appreciate the significance of the fantasies and unconscious thoughts about life in the womb late in life. They contain both the explanation for the strange fear of so many people of being buried alive, as well as the deepest unconscious justification of the belief in life after death, which is only the projection into the future of this uncanny life before

birth. Incidentally, the act of birth is the first experience of fear and thus the source and model of the fear effect.

(S. Freud: The Interpretation of Dreams, 3rd edition, 1908, p. 405)

Through these clarifications, however, a deeper layer of experience became accessible, namely that of primary pre-linguistic self-organisation and self-discovery and the associated primordial force in the field of the maternal relationship. Their positive aspects were summarised by Jung (1912, 1985) in the metaphor of an archaic self and the archetypal forces from a maternal primordial ground and their negative aspects were summarised by Adler (1907) as primary damage, inferiority complex and compensatory power drive.

Both therefore already had the prenatal dimension in mind, but this could only be hinted at at the time.

(Janus 2021b, p. 1)

The conceptual break between Freud and Rank can now be precisely understood thanks to the publication of their correspondence. In a letter dated 15 February 1924, Freud wrote of the "womb fantasies", to which Rank had only given a special meaning. On the same day, Rank replied that he felt misunderstood here, that he was concerned with the "reality of the womb"

(Janus 2021b, p. 2).

It is historically significant and also regulating from a historical perspective that, after Freud had explored the male-paternal dimension of our life history, it was of elementary value to obtain an analytical exploration of the female-maternal dimension of our life history and its hidden significance in cultural history in Rank's book.

But the great difficulty in therapy is that the immaturity of the parents or the unwanted nature of a pregnancy is one of the most difficult issues. Any form of devaluation of families, couples and individual existences must be avoided at all costs. And the therapist is also confronted with these deep questions themselves and must face them in their own self-awareness in order to be able to accompany other people responsibly. "Accepting the reality of prenatal development and the birth experience can often mean a shattering self-confrontation with one's own unwantedness and endangerment on a very elementary level" (Janus 2014, p. 6).

Due to the resistance of the psychoanalytic community and social opposition, further research was often continued by individual doctors and psychoanalysts with strong personalities, who were less fixated on authority and fearful, trusted their own observations in practice and the statements of their patients more and also published this.

The pioneers and their most important publications

Sandor Ferenczi makes the first psychological attempt at a systematic description of prenatal development. Based on his psychoanalytical, medical and intuitive practice, he examines the drive and need structures of each stage in a specific sequence of prenatal development, whereby the child gains an image of reality that is further developed postnatally.

Developmental Stages of the Sense of Reality 1913
Attempt at a Genital Theory 1924

Otto Rank: *The Trauma of Birth*

> Birth is the primal trauma, the primal disturbance that underlies all later disorders. An intact, functioning system is traumatised for the first time by the birth process. Every fear is based on fear of birth and every desire ultimately tends to restore intrauterine lust.

The Trauma of Birth 1924, p. 20
Technique of Psychoanalysis 1927, 1929 and 1931

Gustav Graber: The trauma of birth consists less in the birth process than in the "change of the mode of existence". The "primal resistance" of the human being consists in the Refusal to accept a psychic experience before birth: "All our scientific and psychotherapeutic endeavours to understand the human".

The Integration of Prenatal Life into the Biography and Patho-graphy of the Personality (Blurb 1978)
The Ambivalence of the Child 1924
Collected Writings 1978

In 1924, the midwife and paediatric nurse **Dorothy Garley** published her report "On the Shock of Being Born and Its Possible After-Effects" (Garley 1924) in the *International Journal of Psychoanalysis* (ed. Freud).

She is one of the first women to write on pre- and perinatal topics. She empathises directly with the child itself during the birth process and criticises the denied emotional dimension of birth in healthcare: obstetricians

> Are satisfied if the child emerges from the womb physically undamaged. And yet the emotional repercussions of the experiences during birth are of at least as great, one could even say greater, significance for a human being in the process of becoming than the physical ones.

> *(Garley 1924 p. 135)*

Anna Freud is of the opinion that intrauterine experience in the actual cannot be the object of analytical endeavour. In the spirit of her father, who sharply distanced himself from Rank after his initial enthusiasm, she propagates a demarcation of psychoanalysis operating in the field of postnatal object occupations from an "oceanic feeling" of prenatal unity reality time. However, the following sentence has been handed down from her: "…in my opinion, these oldest environmental influences create conditions that are comparable to deficiency diseases on the physical side" (Schindler 1983).

Nandor Fodor was one of the first to describe very clear connections between prenatal and postnatal psychodynamics and postnatal illnesses of all kinds. His student **Francis Mott** continued this work.

N. Fodor: *The Search for the Beloved* 1949
F. Mott: *The Nature of the Self* 1959

Wilhelm Reich's work opens up the field of body psychotherapy for the work of prenatal psychology. He was one of the first doctors to set up counselling centres for pregnant women in Vienna and New York. With his vegetotherapy developed from 1934 onwards, Reich laid the foundation for body psychotherapy, which his student **Alexander Lowen** expanded on in bioenergetics.

Michael Balint: The basic disorder ("lack of fit") lies in the incompatibility of the parents.
Balint follows on from Ferenczi. *Primary Love* is a pre-ambivalent form of object relationship, a prenatal object relationship. In its original form, primary love is a harmonious entanglement with an undifferentiated environment, a world of primary substances. The discovery that in the primary love "vital parts are independent and inscrutable is traumatic, but has a structure-creating effect…This discovery turns the world into solid, resistant objects, between which there are separating intermediate spaces" (Balint *Primary Love* 1952, p. 5).

Primary Love 1952
The Basic Fault 1968

Frank Lake:
In England, Frank Lake was able to specify the consequences of prenatal and birth traumatisation.

Lake worked with LSD 25 from 1954 to 1969 when he began using also a method of deep breathing. The insights Lake gained into the mother-fetal effects were to be corroborated in other fields, sociology and criminology, obstetrics and biochemistry. Lake was encouraged by the earlier discernment of pre- and perinatal influences by Fodor, Peerbolte, Mott, Winnicott and Swartley, and highly critical of Freud's volte-face having first backed Rank's emphasis on the birth trauma. This had seriously delayed primal integration work.

Lake found that the patient must become conscious of the original context of a primal memory, in order to re-integrate the separate memory systems. Working with large num bers, he discovered a convincing common memory of the complete primal journey. He led patients through the primal journey so they each could explore their own pre- and perina tal experiences. He defended scientifically the feasibility that cell memory could antedate brain memory, quoting his own research and also that of Dryden and Pribram.

(House 1999, p. 437)

With Respect 1982
In the Spirit of Truth 1991

Melanie Klein, Rene Spitz, John Bowlby and Margarete Mahler focus their work on the early postnatal bond between mother and child and express cautious or clearly differentiated views on the psychological experience of an intrauterine bond. **Daniel Stern** also focuses exclusively on the postnatal development of the self (D. Stern: *The Interpersonal World of the Infant*, 1985).

J.A. Caruso: "Caruso is one of the co-founders of the first professional association "International Study Group for Prenatal Psychology (ISPP)" in 1971 and one of the first presidents after Graber. In his book *Narcissism and Socialisation* (1976), he describes the need for a healthy emotional economy in the mother/child dyad in the prenatal and postnatal period. Prenatal trauma and postnatal rejection are a heavy burden for the formation of a healthy sense of self and trust in the world" (Janus 2000, p. 88).

Narcissism and Socialisation 1976

Kruse, Rascovsky, Garma, Peerbolte work on the scientific basis of the continuity of the self from conception to death.

Ronald Laing: He was one of the first psychiatrists to notice that patients who lay naked on the floor in their cell or in the group room of a psychiatric ward in the foetal position and are no longer responsive are in a deep regression, that it is about memories of being exposed, unprotected even in the womb, with the hope that someone will recognise it and develop understanding. In other words, these "productions" indicate a field of memory and are not just a dissocial provocation.

The Facts of Life 1982

Donald Winnicott endeavours in vain to promote a stronger international discussion on prenatal psychology. In his work *Birth Memories, Birth Trauma and Anxiety* (1949), Winnicott states that "there is evidence that the personal birth experience is significant and can be fixed as memory material", and he emphasises that "there is no such thing as the treatment of birth trauma alone" (1949).

Birth Memories, Birth Trauma and Anxiety 1949

Artur Janov: Janov developed his method to activate pre-linguistic feelings and body sensations by intensifying breathing and to find access to traumatic experiences of birth and the prenatal period.

The Liberated Child 1977
Early Imprints 1984

Stanislav Grof: Grof used LysergSäureDiethylamid (CAS-Nr. 50-37-3) (LSD) and other psychoactive substances to enable patients to access pre-linguistic experiences. This enabled Grof (1983) to systematise the birth process into four matrices: the phases of unity, opening, expulsion and emergence. He observed the connections between this existential experience and basic dynamic for all people in therapeutic and cultural-historical processing.

Topography of the Unconscious 1983

Edeltrud Meistermann-Seeger: "Man's first relationship, even if it is only a germ, is with his parents". In her Balint-orientated extension of the focal therapy, it is about formulating the basic deficiency of a person that arises from the incompatibility of the parents. The talent and conflict patterns of an ontogenesis lie in this incompatibility. Through deep regressive work, a person's own decision for one's own life is consciously renewed, confirmed and recognised.

Short Therapy Focal Training 1989

Lloyd DeMause: The American historian and psychohistorian opens the discourse on the prenatal causes and conditions of historical processes.

Foundations of Psychohistory 1982

Hans Carl Leuner initiated the "European Collegium for Altered States of Consciousness" as a forum for research into pre-linguistic and prenatal borderline perceptions of consciousness. He developed catathymic imagery as a therapeutic method.

Hallucinogens 1981

Francoise Dolto: The infant cannot speak but can understand speech.

The French psychoanalyst works with infants in orphanages and achieves significant success in curing psychosomatic symptoms by talking to the children and explaining their life situation, also with reference to the prenatal period.

La cause des enfants 1985

Sepp Schindler: The Salzburg developmental psychologist worked on the developmental psychology of the prenatal period. He held a chair in psychology at the University of Salzburg.

Ecology of the Perinatal Period 1983

Athanassios Kafkalides: The work of the Greek psychiatrist and psychotherapist Athanassios Kafkalides, *The Knowledge of the Womb* (1995), was groundbreaking for the understanding of prenatal trauma.

Thomas Verny: Verny works on the psychobiology of the prenatal period and was able to publish an international bestseller with the book *Das Seelenleben des Ungeborenen* in 1981.

The Soul Life of the Unborn Child 1981
The Embodied Mind 2021

W.E. Freud: Freud's favourite grandson became a psychoanalyst himself and conducted research on premature baby wards in hospitals. He was an important advocate of the "perinatal continuum", i.e. the primary importance of physical contact between premature babies and the mother and father, the kangaroo method.

Collected Writings 2000

Peter Fedor-Freybergh: Professor of Neurology in Stockholm, Prague and Bratislava. The psychoneuroendocrinology of pregnancy and birth makes it possible to clarify biopsychological relationships about the first human biotope. He is the editor of the first journal for prenatal psychology: *The International Journal of Pre- and Perinatal Psychology and Medicine*, 1989 ff. President of the ISPPM until 1995.

Prenatal and Perinatal Psychology and Medicine 1988

Ludwig Janus: The new research findings of prenatal psychology do not require a break with the psychoanalytical tradition but rather a new understanding of its interpretation. The Heidelberg doctor and psychoanalyst has published over 250 scientific papers on prenatal psychology and was President of the "International Research Association for Pre- and Perinatal Psychology and Medicine" (ISPPM) from 1995 to 2005. He is the most comprehensive theorist of prenatal psychology worldwide and, following on from Lloyd DeMause, also explores the cultural-theoretical and psychohistorical contexts of prenatal psychology. He is co-editor of the specialist journal *International Journal of pre- and perinatal Psychology and Medicine* 1989 ff.

How the Soul Is Created 1993
The Psychoanalysis of the Prenatal Period and the Birth 2000
Handbook of Prenatal Psychology 2021

William Emerson and his student Karlton Terry are pioneers in the field of baby therapy and birth trauma therapy. The body therapy setting with its emphasis on sensations and feelings proved to be particularly suitable for making the pre-linguistic level of prenatal and birth experience accessible.

Emerson W. *Birth Trauma* 2017
Terry K. *From Crying to Cuddling, from Crying to Bliss. Understanding and Healing Babies* 2014

Alessandra Piontelli: Long-term studies from ultrasound observation of the foetus to the five-year-old child show significant consistent analogies of behavioural patterns.

From Fetus to Child 1992

Helga Blazy: The German psychotherapist and cultural researcher popularised attachment analysis in Germany and researches ethnological references to prenatal psychology.

How to Hear an Inner Voice – Bonding in the Prenatal Space 2009

Ray Castellino: Castellino developed the "Womb Surround" concept. He developed care principles and specialised training to understand the earliest layers of experience and promote family work and understanding of the baby's implicit world.

Consciously Parenting 2004

Joanna Wilheim: The South American psychoanalyst analyses transgenerational and prenatal imprinting. The basic material of the unconscious begins, at the latest, at conception. The transgenerational transmission of traumatic experience, among other things, is not limited to biochemical language games (genetics). It works on the foundation of a pre- and periconceptual psychology.

On the Way to Birth 1995

Lloyd DeMause: The American historian establishes psychohistory as a specialised science that applies the findings of prenatal psychology to the study of history.

The Emotional Life of Nations 2005

Peter Sloterdijk: With his Spheres trilogy, the German philosopher establishes an opening of philosophy to prenatal psychology.

Spheres 1–3 1998 ff

Jenö Raffai: No freedom without attachment. Through intrauterine contact with the mother, the child begins to perceive itself more clearly as an independent being. Through his work with schizophrenic patients, the Hungarian psychoanalyst discovered aetiological connections with pregnancy. He establishes mother-child attachment analysis as psychological support and promotion of mother-child contact during pregnancy.

The Greater Development Opportunities of the Child in the Mother-Body Through Attachment Analysis 1999
The Umbilical Cord of the Soul 2006

Franz Renggli: The Swiss doctor and psychoanalyst works on systemic issues and deals with prenatal trauma with families, couples and babies. He also works on psychohistorical issues.

Early Experiences – The Key to Life. How Our Traumas from Pregnancy and Birth Can Heal 2018

Rupert Linder: The gynaecologist and psychotherapist founded psychosomatic pregnancy care. Founder of the Pforzheim Study, a long-term study on transgenerational relationships. Pregnancy-related work that helps to recognise and resolve stress from the individual and family past by integrating medical, psychotherapeutic and social levels, thereby increasing individual resilience. It has been proven that this has significantly improved obstetric events. In the Pforzheim study currently being conducted (together with Gerlinde Metz), these relationships are being analysed in detail from a psychological and obstetric point of view, including metabolomic and epigenetic control. He is co-editor of the *Lehrbuch für Pränatale Psychologie* and the *Handbook of Prenatal Psychology*.

Handbook of Prenatal Psychology 2021

Klaus Evertz: The artist and therapist developed "integrative art and body therapy" and "analytical-aesthetic art therapy", forms of therapy that are prenatally based and integrate prenatal patterns through painting and body experience. He is founder of "prenatal aesthetics", which ultimately explains all aesthetic qualities in art from the early body and emotional experiences of ontogenesis, which are always bonding and relationship experiences from the moment of conception. In their psychohistorical functions, the arts therefore always also contain pre- and perinatal and early postnatal transitional object levels. He is editor of the *Lehrbuch für Pränatale Psychologie* and the *Handbook of Prenatal Psychology*.

Art Analysis 2002
Textbook for Prenatal Psychology 2014
Handbook of Prenatal Psychology 2021

Kate White: The American physiotherapist Kate White has developed a comprehensive low-threshold training programme to deal with pre- and perinatal attachment trauma. She is a member of APPPAH, the American Association for Prenatal Psychology.

Olga Guni: The Greek prenatal therapist organised the World Congress in October 2023: Prenatal Sciences Global Congress https://www .prenatalsciencespartnership.org

There are many other pioneers without whom the field of prenatal psychology could not have developed. It is impossible to mention them all here (see also Janus 2000, 2021).

The medical-epidemiological and psychobiological strands of research developed partly independently of the tradition of prenatal psychology and are described in Chapter 3.

Summary

Prenatal psychology, which deals with the psychological development of the foetus and the interaction between the unborn child and its environment, has gone through various stages of development throughout history. Here is an initial chronological list of the historical development of prenatal psychology:

1 Early cultures: In many early cultures, there were already ideas that the unborn child is influenced by the experiences and emotions of the mother and father, as well as the ancestors. These ideas were often shaped by spiritual or religious beliefs and were celebrated and honoured in rituals. In many cultures, the "celebration of life" was already prepared pre-conceptually with songs, dances, poetry and other forms of art, and the young girl and young man were attuned to their roles as future mother and future father.

2 During the Enlightenment, there were a number of authors and doctors who pointed out the connection between prenatal life and the fate of human beings, such as Johann Karl Wezel:

> It was therefore noted that it would be very easy to explain not all, but most of the currently inexplicable phenomena that appear in many people to the astonishment of scholars and unscholars, if someone made known an exact and detailed history of their fates in the womb from the first moment of their existence until their birth.
>
> *(Janus 2014, p. 5)*

3 With advances in medical science in the 19th century, some psychologically interested researchers began to explore the idea that prenatal experiences could influence the child's later development. Sigmund Freud was one of the first to suggest the importance of prenatal experiences in his psychoanalytic theories. His students Sandor Ferenczi, Otto Rank and Wilhelm Reich, as well as Karl Gustav Graber and others, developed this idea much more clearly in the first half of the 20th century. Nandor Fodor published "The Search for the Beloved: A Clinical Investigation of the Trauma of Birth and Pre-Natal Conditioning" in 1949. He and his student Francis Mott marked the beginning of prenatal psychology even more clearly.

4 In the 1960s, researchers such as Winnicott, Grof, Janov, Verny and Chamberlain began to investigate the role of prenatal experiences on the psychological development of the child. They emphasised the importance of the prenatal environment for later personality development (Janus 2000).

5 Late 20th century: With advances in technology such as ultrasound and foetal monitoring, researchers were able to learn more about the behaviour and reactions of the unborn child. This led to a growing interest in prenatal psychology and the influence of prenatal experiences on later development. Long-term studies such as the one by Alessandra Piontelli were carried out to observe children from pregnancy to school age. Michel Odent and Frederic Leboyer endeavoured to improve the birth culture in industrialised countries and propagated "gentle birth". In her book *Vita activa*, the philosopher Hannah Arendt expands on the idea that life must be thought of from the beginning and not, as the predominantly patriarchal history of philosophy has interpreted life in terms of death. Ludwig Janus became the most important internationally active theorist of prenatal psychology. Following Arendt, Peter Sloterdijk opens up a philosophy of the prenatal (Sloterdijk 1998). Thomas Verny opens up the holistic perspective of embodiment for the whole of life from conception to death (Verny 2021).

6 Today: Prenatal psychology has become a transdisciplinary field that integrates findings from areas such as developmental psychology, neuroscience, medicine and social sciences. There continues to be

bio-psycho-social research on the influence of prenatal experiences on the cognitive, emotional and social development of the child as well as on ways to support expectant parents during pregnancy. In 2021, the *Handbook of Prenatal and Perinatal Psychology* by Evertz, Janus and Linder will be published as the first global summary of the most important findings in prenatal psychology (Evertz et al. 2021).

This very abbreviated historical development shows how the understanding of prenatal psychology has evolved over time and how it is now recognised as an important field within psychology.

The journals of scientific prenatal research

- *International Journal for Prenatal and Perinatal Psychology and Health* from 1989 to 2012. Digitised at www.mattes.de.
- *Journal of Prenatal and Perinatal Psychology and Health*, www.birth-psychology.com.
- *La Revista Italiana di Educazione Prenatale e alla Genitorialita*, www.anep.it.
- *Il Giornale Italiano di Psychologia e di Educazione Prenatale*, www.anpep.it.

Overviews

Egloff G, Djordjevic D (eds.) (2019) *Pre- and postnatal psychology and medicine*. Nova Science, New York.

Evertz K, Janus L, Linder R (2014) *Textbook of prenatal psychology*. Mattes, Heidelberg.

Evertz K, Janus L, Linder R (eds.) (2021) *Handbook of prenatal psychology*. Springer, New York.

Janus L (2022) *The psychological dimension of pregnancy and birth*. Mattes, Heidelberg.

Janus L (2024a) *How the soul is created. Our psychic life before, during and after birth*. Expanded new edition. Mattes, Heidelberg.

Janus L (2024b) *Enduring effects of prenatal experiences – Echoes of the womb*. Cambridge Scholars Publishing, Cambridge.

Ridgway R (2006) *The unborn child*. Karnac, London, New York.

Literature

Evertz K, Janus L, Linder R (eds.) (2021) *Handbook of prenatal psychology*. Springer, New York.

Ferenczi S. (1913) "Entwicklungsstufen des Wirklichkeitssinnes". In: Ferenczi S, *Bausteine zur Psychoanalyse*, Band 1. S. 62–83. Huber, Bern 1964.

Ferenczi S, Rank O (1924) *Entwicklungsziele der Psychoanalyse. Zur Wechselbeziehung von Theorie und Praxis*. Turia & Kant, Wien (1995).

Fodor N (1949) "The traumata of the unborn". In: Fodor N (Hrsg) *The search for the beloved. A clinical investigation of the trauma of birth and the prenatal condition*. University Books, New York, 303–382.

Garley D (1924) "Über den Schock des Geborenwerdens und seine möglichen Nachwirkungen". In: *Internationale Zeitschrift für Psychoanalyse* X(2): 134–164. Verfügbar auf: https://www.pep-web.org/document.php?id=izpa.010.0134a

Hidas G, Raffai J (2006) *Die Nabelschnur der Seele*. Psychosozial, Gießen.

House S (1999) "Primal integration therapy – School of Lake". In: *International Journal of Prenatal and Perinatal Psychology and Medicine* 11(4): 437–457.

Janus L (2000) *Die Psychoanalyse der vorgeburtlichen Lebenszeit und der Geburt*. Psychosozial, Gießen.

Janus L (2013) "Überlegungen zum wissenschaftlichen Status der Psychodynamischen Psychologie". In: *Psychodynamische Psychotherapie* 12: 61–69.

Janus L (2014) "Die Geschichte der Pränatalen Psychologie". In: Evertz K et al. (eds.) *Lehrbuch der Pränatalen Psychologie*. Mattes, Heidelberg, 3–11.

Janus L (2021a) "The history of prenatal psychology". In: Evertz K et al. (eds.) *Handbook of prenatal psychology*. Springer, New York, 3–8.

Janus L (2021b) *Freud und die pränatale Dimension des seelischen Erlebens*. Unveröffentlicht.

Janus L (2023) "Otto Rank. Der verstoßene Begründer der psychoanalytischen Objektbeziehungspsychologie". In: Abel T (Hg.) *Handbuch der Objektbeziehungspsychologie*. Psychosozial, Gießen, 59–74.

Rank O (1924) *Das Trauma der Geburt und seine Bedeutung für die Psychoanalyse*. Psychosozial, Gießen (1998).

Schindler S, Zimprich H (1983) Ökologie der Perinatalzeit. Hippokrates, Stuttgart.

Sloterdijk P (1998ff) Sphären 1-3. Suhrkamp, Stuttgart.

Verny T (2021) *The embodied mind*. Pegasus, New York.

Whitebook J (2018) *Freud – Sein Leben und Denken*. Cotta, Stuttgart.

3

TRANSGENERATIONAL AND PRENATAL PROGRAMMING

Scientific research

Scientific research in recent decades has produced a wealth of knowledge about the genetic and epigenetic programming of humans. Transgenerational transmission of happiness and suffering, biologically speaking, including oxytocin potentials and stress patterns, and the epigenetic modification of genetic inheritance in the intrauterine phase are now well documented. Consideration of the effects of transgenerational and prenatal stress on life-long health is now crucial for improving strategies to promote healthy development and successful ageing. The contributions of international research on Developmental Origins of Health and Disease (DOHaD), for example, provide comprehensive information on the importance of a healthy genetic inheritance and a healthy pregnancy and on the need to prevent high-risk pregnancies. DOHaD research is based on epidemiological data, followed by clinical, experimental and epigenetic studies. They show that pre- and peri-natal events have a major influence on peri- and postnatal development and on the development of diseases in childhood, adolescence and adulthood (Van den Bergh 2014, 2021; Van den Bergh et al. 2017). For health policy, this means that the more that is invested in the prevention of early disorders and impairments, the lower the likelihood of illness in later life and the lower the healthcare costs (Figure 3.1).

Prenatal psychology mediates between scientific knowledge and a person's world of feelings and emotions. Here, bridges can be built between medical diagnoses and a person's own understanding of themselves and the world but especially to the inner knowledge of each person about their own vitality and their origins in their family system. A wealth of therapeutic documentation shows how a person's inner knowledge and feelings can coincide with biological-medical descriptions (see also Chapters 6–9).

DOI: 10.4324/9781003480242-3

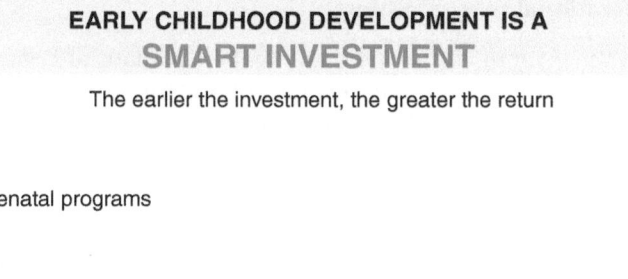

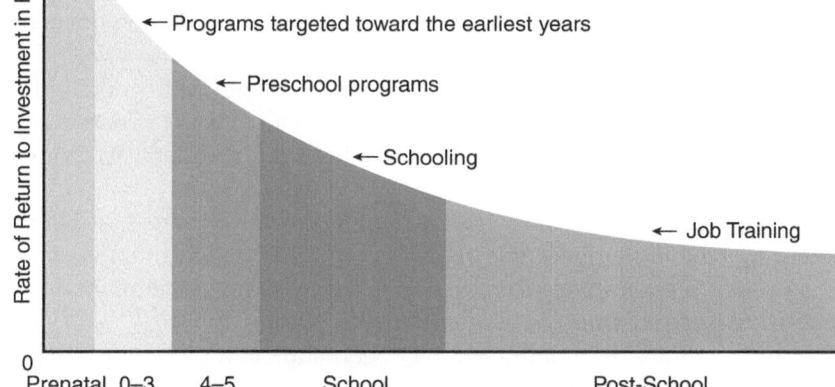

FIGURE 3.1   The earlier investment is made in the safe development of a child, the more it pays off in terms of social healthcare costs.

In medical-epidemiological research, the realisation developed that the prenatal environment to a certain extent predetermines the basis of the physiological control of the organism. The extensive corresponding research is summarised under the heading of "fetal programming" and is now so advanced that empirical studies on prenatal influences are available for almost all significant disease areas. The titles of the basic works "The Fetal Matrix: Evolution, Development and Disease" (2004) and "Developmental Origins of Health and Disease" (2006) by the Australian/English epidemiologists Peter Gluckman and Mark Hanson directly express the claim to scientific explanation. In Germany, this new research was summarised again in the book "Perinatal Programming - State of the Art" (2011) edited by Andreas Plagemann. In her work "Prenatal programming of cognition and emotion: From birth to age 20", the Dutch stress researcher Bea Van den Bergh builds a direct bridge from epidemiological research to prenatal psychology. It describes the basic neurophysiological processes in the prenatal pre-imprinting of thinking, feeling and behaviour.

(Janus 2014, p. 7)

Transgenerational programming

It is about the exciting topic of the fact that all humans are part of a chain of humans and, in evolutionary terms, part of a chain of living beings that has been unbroken for hundreds of millions of years. From this perspective, all living humans are actually "eternal". Because each individual would not exist if this chain had been interrupted somewhere. If you go back just 300 years, i.e. an average of ten generations, each person has 1024 ancestors. From this huge gene pool, it is a matter of condensed life experiences that are passed on. So of course there is a bio-psycho-social connection between the generations, and the last three generations in particular are generally known in the family novel, at least the conspicuous experiences of fate, both good and bad. There are family systems that significantly pass on all kinds of talents and gifts across generations, such as doctors, artists, theologians, scientists, craftsmen and farmers.

However, global research interest is mainly focused on stress and traumatisation. It is therefore about the transmission of information that is effective and has been proven in animal experiments over many generations but can also be proven for humans in epidemiological studies.

Transgenerational traumatisation has been sufficiently proven biochemically and psychologically!

> Scientists in Constance have shown that severe stress actually modifies the genome: When pregnant women are mistreated by their partners, the gene for so-called glucocorticoid receptors, the molecular sensors that recognise stress hormones such as cortisol and mediate further reactions of the brain like a switching station, is permanently altered in their children.
>
> *(Koch 2012 p. 127)*

- "The mother's body signals to these children that they will grow up in a threatening environment", surmises the Constance psychologist Thomas Elbert, "in later life these children are more anxious and less curious, their stress axis is more susceptible than that of other people" (Koch 2012, p. 127).

At the 19th International Congress of the APPPAH, 3–6 December 2015, Berkeley, California, Thomas Verny spoke of a "common field theory of memory and social epigenetics". It's not the genes that make us, it's the gene expression! However, gene expression varies depending on how we live and how our ancestors lived. Verny emphasised the term "social epigenetics":

- Memory is by no means only bound to the neurones of the cerebral cortex.
- Other body cells can also have memory functions.

- There are memory phenomena in many unicellular organisms, including gametes and immune cells.
- There are many examples of this from simple organisms (e.g. the Archaea) or bacterial communities (Verny 2015).

Assmann not only provides a wealth of evidence for intergenerational inheritance in animal models but also a growing body of evidence for humans.

> Intergenerational inheritance refers to the transmission from parents to children or grandparents to grandchildren, where the germ cells were exposed before conception. For example, there are a considerable number of studies on pollution (Sen et al., 2015), metabolic and atopic diseases (Illum et al., 2018, Knudsen et al., 2018) and some on trauma effects (Yehuda & Lehrner 2018).
>
> *(Assmann 2021, p. 176)*

> According to a 2018 review by Yehuda & Lehrner, research on intergenerational trauma sequelae began with the discovery of clinical behavioural abnormalities in children of Holocaust survivors. Initially, observational studies showed an increased prevalence of post-traumatic stress disorder (PTSD) in children of parents with PTSD. This was followed by reports of biological correlates: children of parents with a trauma background showed altered activity of the HPA axis. Epigenetic studies then investigated corresponding gene regions and found correlations between parental PTSD and methylation patterns in their children.
>
> *(Yehuda et al. 2014, 2016)…*

> In summary, it can be said that transgenerational transmission in humans has been documented on an epidemiological level and in animal models also on a molecular level. In addition, the first molecular epigenetic data for intergenerational inheritance from parents to children are now also available for humans.
>
> *(Assmann 2021, p. 176 f)*

In a bio-psycho-social scientific field such as prenatal psychology, we assume that human reality is indivisible in the transition of conception, the merging of the two hereditary genes of father and mother. The scientific divisions into biology and psychology, as valuable as they are, are only models of reality but not reality itself. The family-systemic conditions of the paternal and maternal family and the quality of love between man and woman are already a psychic structure and decisive for the psychic developmental possibilities of the new human being. The biologically describable substrate and the psychologically describable (and memorable) circumstances are models of the attempt to fully understand human reality. Every human being as an individual therefore begins in conception and ends with death.

A "pre-existence of the soul" therefore "only" exists in the bio-psycho-social conditions of the family system and the ancestors that led to its conception. However, the fact that this is a tremendous (information) wealth is often overlooked. A "post-existent soul" can therefore only exist as a legacy of a person's deeds, feelings and thoughts in their descendants and/or in their works and in all their social relationships. As a rule, this is also a great wealth.

> Eternity is,... that the life of every person who has ever lived and will ever live must also be lived, from the beginning to the end says the Dutch writer Margriet de Moor.

Gerlinde Metz, who conducts research in Canada at the University of Lethbridge, Alberta, has gained insights in her scientific studies into how stressful life experiences, particularly during pregnancy, affect subsequent generations. It seems particularly remarkable that not only the genes are inherited but also the information about whether the cells should use these genes or not and how epigenetics modifies gene expression during pregnancy (Babenko 2015; Metz & Hoover 2021; Yao 2014).

Metz analyses the following questions:

– What impact can this have on future generations?
– What conclusions does this mean for working with pregnant women and young families?
– What are the transgenerational effects of prenatal stress?
– What possibilities for prevention do these new findings from epigenetics open up for early prophylaxis and child protection in youth and health care?
– How can youth and health services promote resilience and thus mitigate the consequences of transgenerational stress?
– What does this mean for cooperation between healthcare and youth welfare services?

> Our latest research study, *"Ancestral exposure to stress epigenetically programmes preterm birth risk and adverse maternal and newborn outcomes,"* shows that stress in pregnant rats can shorten the length of pregnancy in subsequent generations. The findings could provide clues to the causes of preterm birth in humans... The multigenerational stress lineage resembles generations living in a continuously stressful environment, compared to the short-term stress affecting only one generation. I think this has interesting implications for human populations, such as stress programming by migration, disasters, and poverty.
>
> *(Metz 2014, 2021)*

Periconceptional and prenatal programming

The most sensitive and vulnerable part of our lives is the first two weeks of our lives. About 30 hours after the egg and sperm cell fuse, the cell divides for the first time. Now cell divisions begin to increase rapidly. From the sixth day, implantation in the uterine lining begins. The bladder cyst is now 0.2 mm in size. Now begins a complete restructuring of the embryo, which some biologists and cultural scientists describe as a "dance":

> If one little thing goes wrong during this dance," says biologist Zernicka-Goetz, "the pregnancy fails." Around three out of ten embryos are rejected in the first seven days. A further three embryos do not survive the week after implantation. So around six out of ten pregnancies end before a woman even knows about them, says the biologist, more than half.
>
> *(Schlak 2024, p. 2)*

Biologist Zernicka-Goetz is one of the leading researchers in embryology and cultivates artificial embryos from pluripotent cells.

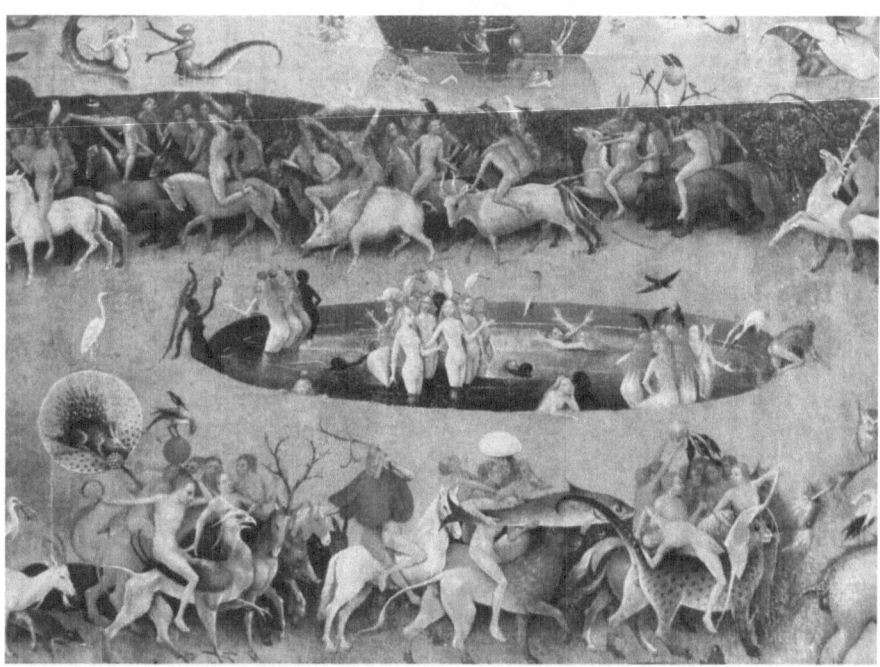

FIGURE 3.2   The painter Hieronymus Bosch painted this "dance" over 500 years ago: *The Garden of Earthly Delights*, detail of centre panel, Prado, Madrid.

It is important for biological research why so many embryos die before and during implantation. And why it is here, in the first two weeks of human life, that the aetiology of many later pre- and postnatal disorders and diseases begins.

In terms of cultural psychology and also prenatal psychology, the fact that almost two-thirds of all pregnancies end at implantation is also very significant. Apparently, the extremely complicated coordination of the female body's immune tolerance with the new cell structure is so fragile that implantation only succeeds and the pregnancy continues if there is a particular match. Prenatal psychology is based on many bio-psycho-social factors that are decisive for the onset of pregnancy and further development (Weatherbee 2024).

The complicated biological processes of immune tolerance and immune defence between mother and child explain very well the diverse positive conditions of successful pregnancies as well as the causes of various pregnancy complications (Ott et al. 2021).

The prenatal psychologist Raffai assumes a biopsychological necessity of a fight for life. The mother denies the foreign cell further development if it is not strong enough to assert itself. Most embryos die here unnoticed. If the fight is only just in favour of the new foreign cell, this is where the biochemical causes of later pregnancy and birth complications as well as postnatal susceptibility to disease lie. If immune tolerance can develop more easily, this is a strong basic condition for a long, healthy life with many resiliences (Raffai 1997).

Prenatal imprints – foetal programming

In the last 30 years or so, the aspect of "foetal programming" has become increasingly important in medical research, culminating in the discussion of a huge paradigm shift: the aetiology of the vast majority of physical and mental illnesses is therefore to be found neither in genetics nor in postnatal risk factors but mostly in the epigenetics of pregnancy (Schwab 2009; Van den Bergh 2014, 2021; Verny 2014).

Schwab formulates this new concept of "foetal programming" as follows:

- "In critical phases of fetal development, epigenetic factors can already represent irreversible predispositions for diseases in later life by permanently modifying the function of physiological systems through a change in gene regulation and gene expression, thereby acquiring pathogenetic significance" (Schwab 2009, p. 14).

The main programming influences are:

- Suboptimal foetal nutrient supply (e.g. due to maternal malnutrition or placental insufficiency).

- Increased foetal stress hormone levels (e.g. due to maternal stress or prenatal betamethasone treatment).

> Elevated fetal cortisol concentrations further induce a permanent desensitisation of glucocorticoid receptors in the hippocampus in the last weeks of pregnancy, when the infant pituitary-hypothalamic-adrenal (HNN) axis matures. This results in a reduced negative feedback of the HNN axis with the consequence of an increased release of cortisol and an increased sensitivity to stress in later life.
>
> *(Schwab 2009, p. 13)*

But these medical facts can also be perceived and felt and, under certain circumstances, can determine a person's entire emotional life for life. These early imprints can be dealt with in psychotherapy (Figure 3.3) (Evertz et al. 2014, 2021).

> The crucial connection between mother and foetus is the placenta. The placenta is a (temporary) organ that forms in the maternal uterus after implantation of the blastocyst (cell stage of embryogenesis around the 5th day after fertilisation) from fetal trophoblast cells and the mother's endometrium. Trophoblasts are the outer cell layer of the blastocyst, the endometrium is the mucous membrane inside the uterus. The placenta serves to continuously supply the embryo or - from the 9th week of pregnancy - the foetus with nutrients and oxygen from the mother's metabolism. The connection between the foetus and placenta is via the umbilical cord.
>
> *(Ott et al. 2021, p. 119)*

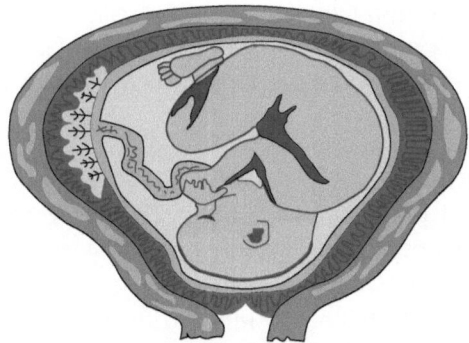

FIGURE 3.3   The connection between the foetus and placenta is via the umbilical cord (Ott et al. 2021, p. 119).

1 Foetal programming refers to the process by which environmental conditions during pregnancy can influence the development and health of the foetus.
2 Studies have shown that foetal programming can have long-term effects on the risk of diseases such as diabetes, cardiovascular disease and obesity in later life.
3 The mother's diet during pregnancy plays an important role in foetal programming and can increase or reduce the risk of metabolic disorders in the child.
4 Other environmental factors such as stress, smoking and alcohol consumption can also influence foetal programming and have long-term effects on the child's health.
5 Foetal programming also has an impact on the child's neurological development and can increase the risk of behavioural disorders and mental illness later in life.
6 With a better understanding of foetal programming, preventive measures can be developed to reduce the risk of disease later in life and improve the health of mother and child (Nathanielz 1999).

A plethora of global studies are contributing to the efforts of interdisciplinary and multidisciplinary researchers investigating the Developmental Origins of Health and Disease (DOHaD) hypothesis. This hypothesis stems from the "fetal programming of adult disease" hypothesis, which states that an unfavourable fetal environment induces plastic responses that increase the risk of chronic diseases such as type 2 diabetes and coronary heart disease later in life. Studies testing the DOHaD hypothesis include early pre- and perinatal origins of a wide range of diseases and disorders, both physical and mental, through unfavourable influences during sensitive periods of development (Gillman 2005; Gluckman and Hanson 2004; Gluckman et al. 2007; Hanson and Gluckman 2014; Nathanielsz 1999; Meaney 2010; Meaney et al. 2007; Phillips and Jones 2006; Seckl 2007; Seckl and Holmes 2007; Schlotz et al. 2008). The DOHaD field of research has been influenced by researchers investigating the adaptive and/or maladaptive nature of neural, physiological and behavioural responses to environmental stressors.

(Van den Bergh 2021, p. 84)

In his book *The Embodied Mind* (Verny 2021), the Canadian psychiatrist, psychotherapist and prenatal psychologist Thomas Verny develops a new view of the foundations of consciousness in bodily experience and the biological intelligence of the body. His holistic perspective aligns with all holistic interdisciplinary psychosomatic and philosophical theories, e.g. the theory of embodiment (see also Chapter 4):

The collective communication and cooperation of the cells is crucial for their effectiveness. Essential parts of the memory are stored in the DNA, but also in the cell membranes and other cell organelles. There is therefore a separate memory system at the level of the body.

Verny quotes Bessel van der Kolk on this: "Your body… remembers everything. The memory… is stored in our body, basally at the cellular level" (Verny 2023). And in view of the interplay between the extremely complex biochemistry of the cells and later the blood circulation and the nerve receptors, the scientist Candace Pert explains: "The body is the unconscious mind!" (House 1999, p. 444).

> The brain does not work in isolation and separately from the body. The neurones of the brain are in constant communication with all other cells, tissues and organs of the body and form an interconnected communication network. The somatic and neuronal memory networks are interconnected and function as a unified system. The brain acts as a transceiver of mental activity, i.e. the mind can act through the brain, but is not necessarily generated by the brain.
>
> *(Verny 2023)*

In terms of scientific and epistemological theory, it should be noted that certain mentalities and experiences are required in order to comprehend these holistic models. Scientists are also predisposed and limited by their personal life experiences and can only understand, achieve and communicate research goals and chains of evidence if their own bio-psycho-social experiences allow this. So in all sciences, the phenomenon of development and progress initially only exists for a few, until the general public can also understand it. How long did it take for the theory of relativity to really be understood by a wider scientific community, despite the given logic and evidence?

(On psychobiology, see also Chapters 4 and 8)–

Literature

Assmann B (2021) "Traces of the invisible world of becoming. Epigenetics as a molecular correlate of prenatal psychology". In: Evertz K, Janus L, Linder R (eds.) *Handbook of prenatal and perinatal psychology*. Springer, New York, S. 169–192.

Babenko O (2015) "Stress-induced perinatal and transgenerational epigenetic programming of brain development and mental health". In: *Neuroscience and Biobehavioral Reviews* 48: 70–91.

Evertz K, Janus L, Linder R (2014) *Lehrbuch der Pränatalen Psychologie*. Mattes, Heidelberg.

Evertz K, Janus L, Linder R (2021) *Handbook of prenatal and perinatal psychology*. Springer, New York.

Gluckman P, Hanson M (2004) *The fetal matrix. Evolution, development and disease*. Cambridge University Press, New York.

Gluckman P, Hanson M (Hg.) (2006) *Developmental origins of health and disease*. Cambridge University Press, New York.

House S (1999) "Primal integration therapy – School of Lake". In: *International Journal of Prenatal and Perinatal Psychology and Medicine* 11(4): 437–457.

Janus L (2014) "Die Geschichte der Pränatalen Psychologie". In: Evertz K et al. (eds.) *Lehrbuch der Pränatalen Psychologie*. Mattes, Heidelberg, 3–11.

Koch J (2012) "Das Leben vor der Geburt". In: *Der Spiegel*, Nr. 25/18.6.2012, 120–128.

Metz G (2014) *University of Lethbridge researchers show that stress during pregnancy has generational effects*. Interview August 2014. UNews, University of Lethbridge.

Metz G, Hoover T (2021) "Transgenerational consequences of perinatal experiences: Programming of health and disease from mother to child and subsequent generations". In: Evertz K et al. (eds.) *Handbook for prenatal psychology – Integrating research and practice*. Springer, Heidelberg, New York, 63–81.

Nathanielz PW (1999) *Life in the womb – The origin of health and disease*. Prometheus Press, Ithaka, NY.

Ott M, Singer M, Bliem HR, Schubert C (2021) "Prenatal psychoneuroimmunology". In: Evertz K, Janus L, Linder R (eds.) *Handbook of prenatal and perinatal psychology*. Springer, New York, S. 115–158.

Plagemann A (2011) *Perinatal programming – The state of the art*. De Gruyter, Berlin, New York.

Raffai J (1997) "Mutter-Kind-Bindungsanalyse im pränatalen Bereich". In: *International Journal of Prenatal and Perinatal Psychology and Medicine* 9(4): 457–466.

Schlak M (2024) "Embryonen aus dem Labor - Die Schöpferin". *Spiegel* 3(24). https://www.google.com/search?client=firefox-b-d&q=Schlak+M+%282024%29+%E2%80%9CEmbryonen+aus+dem+Labor+-+Die+Sch%C3%B6pferin%E2%80%9D.+Spiegel+3%2824%29.

Schwab M (2009) "Intrauterine Programmierung von Störungen der Hirnfunktion im späteren Leben". In: *Gynäkol Geburtshilfliche Rundsch* 49: 13–28.

Van den Bergh BR (2014) "Antenatal anxiety and stress and the neurobehavioural development of the fetus and child: Links and possible mechanisms". In: Evertz K, Janus L, Linder R (eds.) *Lehrbuch der Pränatalen Psychologie*. Mattes, Heidelberg, 70–103.

Van den Bergh BR (2021) "Prenatal developmental origins of early brain and behavior development, of self-regulation in adolescence, and of cognition and central and autonomic nervous system function in adulthood". In: Evertz K et al. (eds.) *Handbook for prenatal psychology – Integrating research and practice*. Springer, Heidelberg, New York, 83–114.

Van den Bergh BR, van den Heuvel MI, Lahti M, Braeken M, de Rooij SR, Entringer S, Schwab M (2017) "Prenatal developmental origins of behavior and mental health: The influence of maternal stress in pregnancy". In: *Neuroscience & Behavioral Reviews* 117: 26–64.

Verny TR (2014) "The pre- and perinatal origins of childhood and adult diseases". In: Evertz K, Janus L, Linder R (Hg.) *Lehrbuch der Pränatalen Psychologie*. Mattes, Heidelberg, S. 50–69.

Verny TR (2015) Lecture: "The common field theory of memory and social epigenetics". *19th International Congress of the APPPAH*, 3–6 December 2015, Berkeley, California.

Verny TR (2021) *The embodied mind. Understanding the mysteries of cellular memory, consciousness and our bodies*. Pegasus Books, New York, London.

Verny TR (2023) Congress promotional flyer: The new format of the scientific-somatic congress, 11/03/2023, TOP Hotel Prague: Thomas Verny about the topic of congress: The embodied mind – The cellular intelligence and memory. S.1.

Weatherbee B (2024) "Distinct pathways drive anterior hypoblast specification in the implanting human embryo". In: *Nature Cell Biology* 26(March 2024): 353–365. https://www.google.com/search?client=firefox-b-d&q=Weatherbee+B+%282024%29+%E2%80%9CDistinct+pathways+drive+anterior+hypoblast+specification+in+the+implanting+human+embryo%E2%80%9D.+In%3A+Nature+Cell+Biology+26%28March+2024%29%3A+353%E2%80%93365.

Yao Y (2014) "Ancestral exposure to stress epigenetically programs preterm birth risk and adverse maternal and newborn outcomes". In: *BMC Medicine*. 12:121, 1–12. http://www.biomedcentral.com/1741-7015/12/121

4

BASIC CONCEPTS OF PRENATAL PSYCHOLOGY

Prenatal psychology (PP) is a transdisciplinary field of research in order to be able to depict the complexity of the human being in a truly scientific and artistic-cultural way. Seven concepts form the theoretical basis of PP:

1 The psychotherapeutic level: The phenomenological-hermeneutic therapeutic research of the prenatal-based depth-psychological schools since Ferenczi and Rank in practice and theory (Janus 2000, 2014, 2021).
2 The nosological level: The bio-psycho-social model (Engel 1980; Ott et al. 2021).
3 The philosophical level: The concept of ontological consciousness (Evertz 2002, 2017, 2021; Evertz et al. 2014, Janus 2016, 2020, Sloterdijk 1998).
4 The anthropological level: The concept of embodiment (Gallagher 2005; Verny 2021).
5 The cultural-anthropological and psycho-aesthetic level: The concept of psychohistory and prenatal aesthetics (Evertz & Janus 2002; Evertz 2017; Janus & Evertz 2008).
6 The psychological level: The concept of prenatal developmental psychology and prenatal attachment theory (Brandon 2009; Evertz 2021; Verdult 2014, 2021).
7 The scientific level: Transgenerational, psychobiological and neuroscientific research on prenatal programming (André 2018; Brandon 2009; Ammaniti & Gallese 2014; Gluckman & Hanson 2004, 2006; Schwab 2009; Plagemann 2011; Evertz 2021; Van den Bergh et al. 2021; Assmann 2021; Metz and Hoover 2021).

DOI: 10.4324/9781003480242-4

The prenatal depth psychology schools, techniques and methods of prenatal psychoanalysis, humanistic psychology, modern art and body psychotherapy, etc. form the enormous empirical background experience of PP. In the context of therapeutic practice, the seven basic concepts of PP form the foundation of today's PP.

The phenomenological-hermeneutic therapeutic research of the prenatal-based depth-psychological schools since Ferenczi and Rank

The prenatal depth psychology schools, techniques and methods of prenatal psychoanalysis, humanistic psychology, modern psychotherapy, art psychotherapy and body psychotherapy, among others, form the enormous empirical background experience of PP.

Everything is a relationship from the very beginning! From the very first cell, the child is in relationship with its entire environment. Even if the child in the first trimester is only understood as a biological entity and only described in biological language, the parents are undoubtedly two adult people who have already had a complex life experience that can be described in bio-psycho-social language and where we have clear evidence that the psychological situation of the parents has a very complex effect on the child, from the very beginning and of course also from their own prehistory, childhood history and transgenerational history. The research conducted in the families of Holocaust survivors over several generations was an important milestone in the transgenerational transmission of experiences of happiness and sadness (Yehuda & Lehrner 2018).

However, PP is not only concerned with the psychological level of the generative transfer of information to the child, but the second level is also research into the child's experiential realities from the very first cell. This raises epistemological, scientific-theoretical and also psychohistorical, psychotherapeutic and psychological questions, which we outline in this chapter. This is about transdisciplinary questions of global culture and research.

In the tradition of psychoanalysis, there is a branch of research that was suppressed from psychoanalysis from 1924 onwards because it focused on precisely this issue: from when does the child have sensations and feelings during pregnancy, and can one remember them in any way, or are there memory patterns in the organism, in behaviour, in thinking and perception or even in pathological developments that can be observed and recognised? Freud already had insights into this dimension of prenatal imprints, but he did not elaborate on them and remained ambivalent. In 1924, his pupil and secretary Otto Rank opened up the perspective of the child's ability to bond, relate and experience even before birth with his book *The Trauma of Birth*. Despite initial enthusiasm, Freud withdrew his approval and Rank was expelled from the Psychoanalytical Association.

His theory "Technique of Psychoanalysis" (Rank 1927, 1929, 1931) was adopted and further developed in the USA by the Humanistic Psychology movement (Janov, Grof, Emerson, etc.) and in England by Lake and Laing (see also Chapter 2).

> The problem in Freud's conceptualisation of the instinctual process is that he sees the independent, instinctively predetermined early childhood needs for food, safety and protection, the need for movement and the need for cleanliness as elements of the sexual need. In doing so, he fails to rec- ognise the autonomy of these instinctive motivations, the satisfaction of which has a completely independent dynamic.
>
> *(Janus 2024, p. 4)*

The error of Freud's drive theory also lies in the fact that he did not separate the healthy and natural drives of eating, drinking, wanting to feel safe and sexuality from the parts of drives to eat, drink, feel safe and have sex, which stem from transgenerational and pre- and perinatal traumatisation. The former can lead to healthy satisfactions, but not the latter. With the former, a healthy level of enjoyment can be maintained, but with the latter, in addition to the possible pleasure, there is always an ultimate feeling of dissatisfaction and remaining unsatisfied, no matter how much you eat, drink or have sex. In the case of the former, lasting peace is achieved after the fulfilment of the drive goal, whereas in the case of the latter, unsatisfied stress persists and even leads to ever-increasing doses of the alleged drive goal, up to and including serious pathological developments such as addictive behaviour or later abuse of all kinds.

Freud was therefore not yet able to distinguish between the strong inner urges and impulses to certain actions, which he called drives, between the healthy instinctive (inner urge) and the dream-generated urge-like states, which could also be described as traumatically deformed impulses or as inner compulsions, the patterns of which can be moulded prenatally. However, both emotional levels feel quite "natural" in an adult, as if they come from one and the same source, just as many patients say: "it has always felt like this" or "it is innate in me" or "it has always been like this, I don't know any other way", because early prenatal trauma and the corresponding imprint- ing could not yet be differentiated theoretically and therapeutically. As it was not possible to differentiate these motivational and behavioural strands therapeutically and theoretically without PP, no clear therapeutic interven- tion for healing early traumatisation could be developed in psychoanalysis, which has contributed to the disappearing importance of psychoanalysis in recent decades, although it has of course achieved epoch-making results in the treatment of exclusively early childhood trauma and the consequences of trauma. Instead of psychoanalysis developing further in terms of developmental psychology, in recent decades it has left the field to behavioural therapists, who are much further away from deep and lasting cures for severe personality disorders. However, the fact that behavioural therapists focus on the urges and fears at the centre of the therapeutic situation means that subsequent integration processes can certainly take place with limited symptoms.

Prenatal traumatisation means such a deep structural disorder that this earliest trauma-generated mixture of strong instinctive impulses with strong trauma-compensatory emergency solution strategies initially appears so "normal" to the person in their psychodynamics and life development that they are unable to recognise the connection with the beginning of their life, even in the case of obvious serious illnesses. Unfortunately, neither do their therapists, which has resulted in many malpractices in psychotherapy in recent decades, even though the relevant knowledge has been available for decades.

The desire for sexuality and the desire for safety and security therefore do not have to contradict each other and come into conflict. Fortunately, passion and family are compatible. They are all the easier to reconcile when a child can experience so much security and love with a father and mother that no contradictions arise. As a rule, these only arise from abuse, abusive projections onto the child, abusive behaviour, narcissistic preoccupation, parentification, excessive demands of all kinds, unresolved traumas in the system, excessive psychosocial stress, etc.

Relationship traumatisation, also through the degree of unhappiness in a couple's relationship from which a child emerges, creates the contradictions between the possibilities of satisfying healthy instincts and unsatisfiable compulsions.

Only prenatal psychotherapy can provide clarification and differentiation about transgenerational, prenatal, perinatal and postnatal trauma and the consequences of trauma (Evertz 2022; Klippel-Heidekrüger & Janus 2022; Janus 2024).

For a long time, dissociative, traumatically generated experiential realities and the resulting dissocial, auto-aggressive and also xeno-aggressive behaviour were understood to be fated. Why do people do something that harms them?

The revision of Freud's drive theory by PP therefore began a hundred years ago. His student Rank therefore already had answers here that he himself did not yet have. A number of psychoanalysts such as Graber, Fodor, Balint, Meistermann-Seeger and Janus continued this revision (Janus 2000, 2024).

To this day, there is extensive therapeutic research on the reality of prenatal experience and when it begins, and which questions are really meaningful

(1) for the psychotherapeutic process and (2) for the human sciences and for a theory of life in general.

In 2021, the *Handbook of Prenatal and Perinatal Psychology* (Evertz 2021) was published as a summary of this research.

(see also Chapters 2, 7 and 12 in particular)

The bio-psycho-social model (Engel 1980)

The bio-psycho-social model is an integrative concept that takes into account the interactions between biological, psychological and social factors in the development and maintenance of health and illness. In the biological area, genetic predispositions, physiological processes and neurological functions are considered. These factors can increase the risk of certain diseases or have protective effects. In the psychological area, individual characteristics such as personality, emotions, ways of thinking and behaviour are taken into account. Psychological factors can influence both the development and progression of diseases. In the social area, environmental factors such as family, friends, work, education and social support are considered. Social factors can have a positive or negative influence on a person's well-being (Figure 4.1).

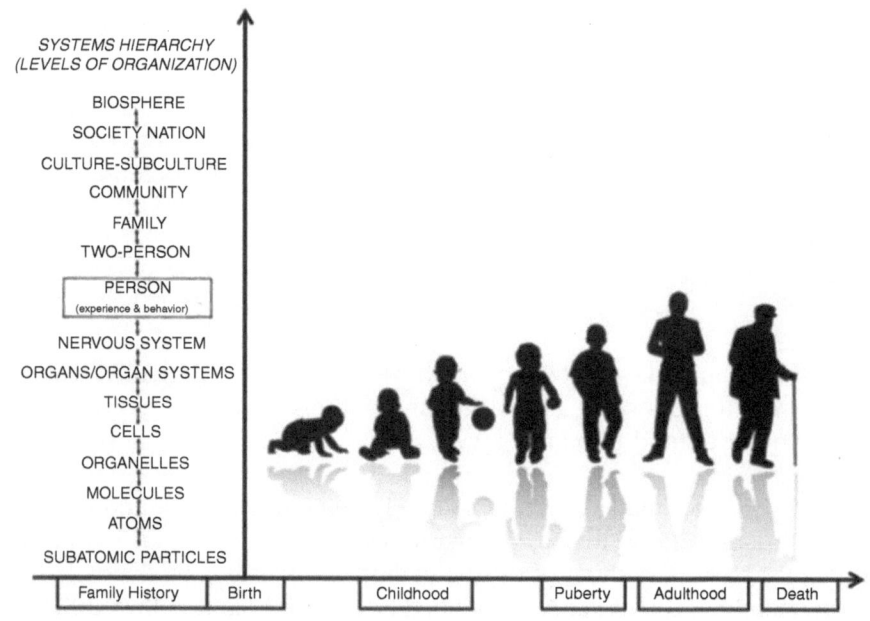

FIGURE 4.1   Bio-psycho-social model Engel 1980. Ott et al. (2021, p. 117).

Psychoneuroimmunology (PNI) investigates the interactions between the psyche, neuroendocrine and immune systems. It thus makes a decisive contribution to the empirical foundation of George Engels' bio-psycho-social model concept. In this model, illness is described as the result of a complex, reciprocal interplay of biological, psychological and social factors, with psychological and social factors being understood as more complex influencing factors.

(Ott et al.2016, p. 144)

Prenatal psychoneuroimmunology (Ott et al. 2021) deepens this research to the prenatal developmental phase:

There is clear scientific evidence that unfavourable environmental influences during prenatal developmental phases are associated with profound and long-term effects on the unborn child. This process is referred to in the specialist literature as "foetal programming" (Barker, et al. 1993; Barker 1998; Huizink et al. 2004; Räikkönen et al. 2011; Seckl et al. 2004; 2007). The intrauterine development phase is characterised by a high degree of sensitivity to environmental and thus also stress influences (Wadhwa 2005). Intrauterine deficiency or overprovision, as well as fetal stress exposure, can lead to misprogramming of organ systems and metabolic processes and thus drastically increase the risk of chronic diseases in adulthood (including obesity, diabetes mellitus, cardiovascular and mental illnesses and cancer) (Plagemann 2005; Beijers et al. 2014; Entringer et al. 2015).

(Ott et al. 2021, p. 118)

PP concretises and expands this model through scientific research into the realities of experience and the bio-psycho-social interrelationships of conception, pregnancy and birth and through therapeutic and psychoeducational practice models (Harms 2017).

The concept of ontological consciousness

In PP, "ontological consciousness" refers to the potential for consciousness, the wealth and abundance of experience and experiential realities that determine the unconscious and consciousness, from the billions of transgenerational, family systemic and biographical influences and information. Whether these are described in biological language (genetic, epigenetic, neurobiological) or in psychological language or in other cultural and scientific languages.

Ontological consciousness, generativity, emergence and embodiment, all four terms denote the same thing in different traditions and different categories: the unity of a human existence as a living system in an evolutionary chain of living systems that, from the first cell until death, functions only as a whole and co-operates on all levels in an unbelievably rich abundance. Emergence means that the smallest particle is capable of change, forms the new network, which in turn is changeable and acts back on the individual particles, which in turn have a permanent effect on the network. Everything that ever happens and will happen to a person, whether as a cell, an embryo, a foetus, an infant, a toddler, a child, an adolescent, an adult or an old person, is perceived and stored by its wholeness and further regulated by it. All perception begins with the first cell. All sensations, feelings and thinking, all perceptions and all behaviours begin there and develop from the transgenerational inheritance and the epigenetic factors, in general from all environmental influences that are ever registered from the cellular and molecular level to the neuronal levels, from nerves, muscles, organs to the CNS, i.e. have an effect, however weak or strong it may be. This is not determinism but a freedom to learn to deal with imprints and find new solutions.

Consequently, all human disorders and diseases have a history and an aetiology that must encompass the entire biography, as well as the transgenerational hereditary potentials and burdens. The biomedical model of disease no longer fulfils the complex demands of modern health policy. We need a comprehensive bio-psycho-social model of illness and health that can creatively alternate the top-down and bottom-up perspectives. The top-down–bottom-up model is a scientific model that is frequently used in various disciplines such as computer science, psychology and management. It describes an approach in which both a superordinate (top-down) and a subordinate (bottom-up) perspective are taken into account.

In the top-down approach, the analysis or planning starts at a higher level and then gradually works its way down to the details. This approach is often used to structure and solve complex problems by first looking at the overall structure before analysing individual parts.

In contrast, the bottom-up approach starts by analysing details or specific observations and then works its way up to an overall structure. This approach is often used to derive new insights from specific observations and then summarise them into a more general theory or explanation.

Capturing the entire history of a person not only biologically, but also psychologically, means that everything experienced can also be remembered and felt if you want to sense and feel it, but illnesses are also memories. Aetiologies describe the development of illnesses, sometimes over years and decades. PP is therefore based on a holistic view of the human being in which nothing of the reality of experience is lost.

In the "field theory" of psychology (Lewin 1963), in the "bio-psycho-social model" according to Engel (Engel 1980), in the considerations of "ontological certainty" according to Laing and Giddens (Elliott 2015), in the model of mirror neurons (Gallese 2013) and many other models of philosophy and psychology, neuroscience and behavioural research, the core question is also whether the constitutional equality of humans as living beings between conception and death does not also mean the potential for a high level of empathy and closeness in interpersonal contact. I call the constitutional certainty of being a living being that consists of the experience of an infinite number of animal and human ancestors "ontological consciousness".

Ontological consciousness as a philosophical term refers to the awareness of the nature of being, existence and reality. It refers to how people perceive and understand the world around them, especially in relation to fundamental questions such as "What is reality?", "What does it mean to exist?" and "What is the nature of reality?"

Ontological consciousness involves the ability to think, feel and sense abstract concepts such as existence, identity, time and space. It is about grasping the essence of things and understanding how they are connected. People with a high level of ontological awareness tend to ask deeper questions about life, the meaning of existence and the nature of reality.

In philosophy and psychology, ontological awareness is often seen as an important aspect of human development. It can help to develop a deeper understanding of oneself, other people and the world around us. By reflecting on ontological questions, people can expand their consciousness and gain new perspectives.

All biological models and psychological models, as well as the philosophical, artistic and religious models of mankind, attempt to describe the reality of human existence. In therapeutic groups, this knowledge is used extensively to overcome crises and develop healing potential for illnesses.

Neither the natural sciences nor the humanities and human sciences have so far been able to offer a stringent theory of life. PP is a key to a theory of life, as it proves a continuous interaction of all living systems and **in all living systems** with the so-called dead matter and the emergence of life and spirit from matter in every ontogenesis of every human being. Thus, every human being actually carries the experience of the transition from matter to consciousness/spirit. The embodied self therefore does not begin after birth, but in the first cell and even there it does not arise completely anew, but from a passing on of the DNA from father and mother, i.e. in a new mixture and formation, but unique. The chain of life is therefore never interrupted. However, if it is never interrupted, the ontological distinction between biology and psychology is no longer tenable, but the heuristic distinction can be maintained where necessary. The distinction between matter and information in a living system is also only superficial. This means that if we understand our first cell, the zygote, the origin of every human being, not only biologically and materially, but also as a corpus of information, intraspecifically and extrospecifically capable of action and reaction, then the concept of "ontological consciousness" is necessary here, because it is the only one that can describe the unity of body and information/spirit/consciousness. Then a happy or unhappy couple in the conception of a child is not only a difference that can be described biochemically, genetically and epigenetically but also a difference that can be described sensitively and emotionally, which will play a fundamental role in human life as primordial happiness or primordial pain.

Memory here does not mean a simple 1:1 form, but a continuous feeling of life, a deep imprint. Memory is not just a neocortical process, nor is it just a process in the amygdala, which already begins to grow in the seventh week of pregnancy but also in the cells that initiate and promote the growth of the amygdala. The basal ganglia cannot simply be remodelled, and severe personality disorders only achieve lasting healing success if the early trauma can be differentiated transgenerationally, periconceptually, prenatally and perinatally! However, this can only be achieved through deep emotional and cognitive therapeutic relationship work, even more successfully with the inclusion of body and art psychotherapy, which takes the earliest human experiences into account.

> Certainly key moments in a child's development are recorded from the very beginning. With appropriate support, the human system can perceive these recordings together with the associated body movements and sensations. Grof called these "condensed experiences" or "COEX systems". The original recording, once stimulated, can resonate with all kinds of similar experiences perceived by the more developed human system, including the brain with its vast memory bank of experiences, stories and vivid scenes.
>
> There is also strong biochemical communication between mother and child, first directly and then via the placenta as development progresses. Lake would certainly have recognised the new understanding of the "wet brain", which functions through biochemical flow even before the brain is "hard-wired". Considering the interplay between the biochemistry of blood circulation and nerve receptors, scientist Candace Pert declares: "The body is the unconscious mind!"
>
> *(House S. 1999, p. 444; Pert 1998).*

The actual spiritual is the body self. Or the spiritual is nothing other than the unconscious body self. "The body is the unconscious mind" (Pert 1998) (House S. 1999, p. 444) – This is the central discovery of PP.

Every person's knowledge of the laws of human existence determines our lives more than the excitement of everyday life shows.

The basic conditions of human life are:

Every human being is born from the encounter between a woman and a man. Every person only has a certain lifespan between conception and death, but this also depends on how they organise their life.

Every person is dependent on all kinds of circumstances in their immediate and wider environment: e.g. on all relationship and bonding conditions, on the natural and cultural environment.

A securely attached child is generally also a wanted child and less at risk of becoming antisocial.

A child from dysfunctional circumstances has a much harder time leading a reasonably good life because it has less inner security and less resilience.

The term "ontological consciousness" therefore describes the potential of awareness possibilities and realities for an entire human life, transdisciplinary. And that the older we get, the more we learn to feel, sense and sense this. For example, the fact that around 2000 chemical reactions take place in our body every second is part of the unconscious knowledge of our physical self. We don't have to consciously control it, it happens on its own.

Embodiment: the embodiment of experience and knowledge

We don't have a body, we are bodies! Our entire feeling and thinking, our entire perception, our behaviour patterns, the functions of our brain, the 2,000 chemical processes that take place in us every second – all of this has grown physically from our first cell. The division into body, soul and spirit is therefore artificial. Embodiment is a concept that deals with the idea that our body is not just a physical vessel but also the only source of knowledge and experience. It is about how we perceive our environment, how we move within it and how these interactions influence our thoughts, emotions and actions.

The term "embodiment" originates from the field of cognitive science and has been increasingly researched in recent decades. It has also gained importance in other fields such as psychology, sociology and philosophy. The concept of embodiment stands in contrast to the traditional dualistic idea of body and mind as separate entities.

A central idea of embodiment is that our body plays a fundamentally active role in the perception and interpretation of our environment. Our senses not only take in information but also process it actively and contextually from the entire history of the organism. This is also much faster in terms of time and always precedes our conscious thinking. The way we move or position our body creates our perception of space and time. When we were a cell, we had our first experiences of movement, of being moved, of opening and closing, of positive and negative environmental factors.

Mind arises from the inner and outer movements and formations of the body in the environment.

One of the pioneers of embodiment, Shaun Galagher, puts it like this:

> For me, the mind is not a substance that you could pin down to a specific place. Rather, the mind is something like the sum of the experiences of my body movements. It develops its form out of my movements in the world.
>
> *(Gallagher 2005)*

But the movements and formations begin with the conception, with the first cell!

One of the pioneers of PP, Frank Lake, wrote back in 1981:

> We have… We have come to the firm conviction that the foetus is vulnerable to everything that goes on in the mother, especially in the first trimester. Suffering in its worst forms strikes in the first three months after conception…. Any severe maternal distress, whatever its cause, is imprinted on the foetus. These damaging experiences are now accessible to consciousness without undue difficulty.
>
> *(House 1999, p. 439)*

Embodiment therefore refers to the way in which our body stores and retrieves knowledge. Our physical experiences and actions are stored in our neuronal memory and in a cellular memory and form the foundation of our perception and thought processes.

Embodiment is a fascinating concept that encourages us to see our body not just as a physical shell but as an active part of our perception, emotions and learning. It opens up new possibilities for research, practice and personal growth. By consciously connecting with our body and using it as a source of knowledge, we can establish a deeper connection to ourselves and the world around us. Other philosophical foundations include the theories of George Herbert Mead, Maurice Merleau-Ponty, Hermann Schmitz and Alfred Schütz's social phenomenology, as well as Peter Sloterdijk.

Prenatal aesthetics – Prenatal theory of sensation and perception

Prenatal aesthetics as an investigation of the sensory qualities and experiential realities in the prenatal space concretises the real level of the initial forms of all our existence. In deeply regressive artistic and therapeutic processes, body psychotherapeutic and art psychotherapeutic, artists and clients can sense and feel their own original conditions in therapeutic processes and thereby differentiate transgenerational, periconceptional and prenatal and postnatal burdens and traumatisation. In this way, sustainable healing can be achieved by mapping the earliest paternal and maternal introjects and relieving the individuality. This is because unresolved parental traumas that have not been mourned cannot be resolved, but this demand is not seen through as a real excessive demand until differentiation is achieved and creates fundamental distress from the outset, which can also be seen in dysfunctional psycho-somatic processes from conception and can manifest itself, for example, in pregnancy complications and birth traumatisation.

- The experiential reality of conception, implantation and pregnancy as the basic aesthetic matrix of all possible images

The aesthetic research of artists has always been concerned with capturing and reflecting patterns of being-in-the-world. In addition to the manifest content, all paintings also carry the latent content of deep regressive knowledge·

The connection between aesthetic and therapeutic culture now gives us a glimpse of the "genetics and epigenetics of aesthetic forms", i.e. we can recognise in the paintings of cultural history not only the respective reflection of historical and social realities but also the developmental processes of individual and collective psychological constitutions.·

All aesthetic forms can ultimately be traced back to physically experienced sensations, feelings and perceptions of the world. Aesthetic archetypes can therefore be traced back to the cell development processes of conception, implantation, prenatal development and birth as bio-psycho-social imprinting events. All art artefacts are not only but always also aesthetic references to pre-linguistic, pre-symbolic, prenatal and periconceptual body memory potentials (Evertz 2002; Janus & Evertz 2008; Evertz 2017, 2021).

The prenatal space of experience, fundamental patterns of world perception, prenatal patterns of perception: see also Chapter 6.

Prenatal development and attachment theory – The prenatal-based model of attachment and relationship

PP forms an extended developmental psychology and an extended attachment theory (Brandon 2009; Verdult 2021; Janus 2024; Evertz 2021).

The deepest human need is to feel a sense of belonging in groups. As part of a group, a person feels strengthened in their self-confidence and wants to contribute to the good of the community. However, the first of all relationships a person has is with their parents, followed by relationships with their family system. The original model of the group is therefore triangulation, i.e. the relationship between father, mother and child. The quality of belonging to this original group is the most important moving force of human existence. The PP examines these qualities of attachment and relationship possibilities.

Prenatal development

1   Prenatal development: This concept refers to the development of the foetus in the womb. It encompasses the various stages of pregnancy and the associated changes in the foetus's body and brain.
2   Prenatal perception: This concept refers to the foetus's ability to perceive various stimuli from its environment. This includes sounds, touch and even taste senses.
3   Prenatal bonding: This concept refers to the emotional bond between the expectant mother and the unborn child. We now know that this bond is formed during pregnancy and has an influence on the later parent–child relationship.
4   Prenatal learning: This concept refers to the foetus' ability to learn and store information from its environment. Studies have shown that babies can recognise certain sounds or voices while still in the womb.
5   Prenatal stress effects: This concept refers to the impact of stress during pregnancy on the unborn child. Research has shown that high levels of stress in the mother can have negative effects on the development of the foetus.
6   Prenatal environmental factors: This concept refers to the various environmental factors to which the foetus is exposed during pregnancy. These include nutrition, smoking, alcohol consumption and environmental toxins, all of which can have an impact on the development of the foetus.
7   Prenatal stimulation: This concept refers to the targeted stimulation of the foetus during pregnancy. This includes, for example, music or gentle touch, which are intended to promote the development of the foetus.
8   Prenatal diagnostics: This concept refers to the various medical tests and examinations carried out during pregnancy to detect possible genetic or developmental problems in the foetus at an early stage.
9   Prenatal intervention: This concept refers to measures that can be taken to treat or prevent potential problems or developmental delays in the foetus. This includes, for example, medical treatments or therapies.
10 Prenatal bonding support: This concept refers to measures and activities aimed at strengthening the bond between the expectant mother and the unborn child. This includes, for example, talking to the baby in the womb or singing songs.

Rien Verdult, a Belgian prenatal psychologist, has created a valuable outline for a prenatal developmental theory that describes the first bonding experiences as the deepest imprint for all later bonds (see Chapter 5).

Love is like "being sadly alone" or love is like "being joyfully in relationship"
Feelings of the mother as a model of love - The central maternal introject

The DNA of the father and mother creates the child. The love of the parents creates the child. Both are correct.

But the growth of the first nine months takes place in the mother. This means that the love of the parents shapes the child with a clear maternal accent. You could also say that the child learns duty (to drive biological growth) from the father and love (the bio-psycho-social forms of this growth) from the mother.

If the mother is doing well during pregnancy and the relationship with the father is also good and sensitive, the mother can welcome the child as a new being through her inner image of the father and through her own well-being and joy and promote its independence The intrauterine child can actually develop and feel its own body boundaries better and perceive itself very early on as its own person with its own identity. This is the best protection in later life to take one's own perception and feelings seriously and not to be easily manipulated. A clear object relationship between parents and their child is actually one of the strongest forms of resilience! (Raffai 2014).

In unhappy relationships, the mother is less able to establish this clear object relationship with the child during pregnancy, as it is difficult to represent the father well. In this case, there is a greater risk that the mother will develop a symbiotic relationship with the child and overburden the child from the outset due to her own needs. The child is supposed to compensate for the mother's feelings of lack, be a substitute partner, fulfil her longings, comfort her or form a coalition with her against the father.

If the father leaves the woman during the pregnancy, this symbiotic pressure can increase. The woman is hurt, feels abandoned and alone, is afraid of the task of perhaps having to give birth and raise the child alone. She is in pain and panic.

These complicated relationship structures in pregnancies always leave their mark on the child for their own later relationship life. For example, a love model of loneliness can develop: Love is being sadly alone. Melancholy or depression can then feel more attractive than real contact with potential romantic partners. It can feel more appealing to sit alone in a café and dream of love than to sit there as a couple and have to organise the relationship, hence the abundance of literature and pop culture about the pain of abandonment and supposedly unattainable love.

Of course, disappointments in love are part of every life course, but people with a stronger identity usually try to learn from them and endeavour to find the next relationship. They do not idealise love relationships but strive for real relationship experiences. Other people with early loss trauma tend to idealise as if there is only one possible partner in the world (the one they have just lost or who is unattainable). These people run the risk of remaining alone or developing a loneliness that repeats the early loneliness without this being reflected upon therapeutically.

Transgenerational, biological, psychobiological and neuroscientific research on prenatal programming

The extensive transgenerational psychobiological and neuroscientific research on prenatal bonding already implies a new understanding of the self that begins in the first trimester. From the very first cell, the human being is a living being that exists continuously in a complex interrelationship with its biotope. There is nothing to prevent us from understanding all of this as forms of bonding, relationships and communication. Or where would one draw the line when it is clear that an unhappy mother is a completely different bio-psycho-social sounding board for the child and its development than a mother who is doing very well? Even the bio-psycho-social qualities of conception, implantation and discovery form fundamental imprints for the child. Today, we can measure and prove this more and more at all levels of research (Ammaniti & Gallese 2014; Gallese 2023; Brandon 2009; Schwab 2009; Plagemann 2011; Ott et al.2021; Gluckman & Hanson 2004, 2006; Van den Bergh 2014; Van den Bergh et al. 2017, 2021; Metz and Hoover 2021).

Ammaniti and Gallese describe the research findings on maternal–foetal bonding for the second and thirrd trimester (Ammaniti & Gallese 2014; Gallese 2023). Why should it be different in the first trimester? The understanding that we are living organisms in permanent exchange with our environment from the very beginning really needs to be thought through to the end. But then our self already begins as a germ, because the sperm and the egg also have a history, whether we describe it only biologically or also psychologically or socially. The first relationship is with the parents, from whose genetic information we are formed, but also from their bio-psycho-social interaction before, during and after conception. From a deep intuitive and aesthetic understanding of ontogenesis, it is sometimes difficult to comprehend how parts of scientific research still persist in a cold, unrelated, mechanistic, technical view of human beings and have no image of a much more permeable bonding atmosphere between father, mother and child, and especially in the maternal–embryonic and maternal–foetal bond. It is as if every event in the mother's life and especially the events experienced before, during and after pregnancy, both in happiness and in suffering, do not have an influence on the child and its entire organism (see also Chapters 3, 7 and 8).

A purely scientific study design is therefore not sufficient to research prenatal bonding, but we must include all cultural and human scientific and therapeutic findings in a transdisciplinary manner if we want to do justice to the totality of human existence and develop a more comprehensive medicine and psychotherapy.

Summary

These seven basic concepts represent the fundamental research levels of PP that are currently being conducted globally in many university institutes, research centres and clinics, as well as in the vast number of psychotherapeutic processes in clinics, practices and psychosocial institutions. Partly in parallel, partly in contact. The task for the future is the further integration of these levels of research and knowledge. Transdisciplinarity always means the ability to link neighbouring but also distant fields of research in human culture and to integrate them in terms of content.

Literature

Ammaniti M, Gallese V (2014) *The birth of intersubjectivity. Psychodynamics, neurobiology and the self.* W. W. Norton & Company, New York.

André V (2018) The human newborn's environment: Unexplored pathways and perspectives. *Psychonomic Bulletin & Review* 25: 350–369.

Assmann B (2021) "Traces of the invisible world of becoming. Epigenetics as a molecular correlate of prenatal psychology". In: Evertz K, Janus L, Linder R (eds.) *Handbook of prenatal and perinatal psychology.* Springer, New York, 169–192.

Brandon A (2009) "History of the theory of prenatal attachment". In: *Journal of Prenatal and Perinatal Psychology Health* Summer, 23(4): 201–222.

Elliott A (2015) *Subject to ourselves: An introduction to Freud, psychoanalysis, and social theory.* Routledge, London.

Engel GL (1980) "The clinical application of the biopsychosocial model". *American Journal of Psychiatry* 137(5): 535–544.

Evertz K (2002) *Kunstanalyse.* Mattes, Heidelberg.

Evertz K (2017) *Das Erste Bild – Pränatale Ästhetik. Schriften zur Kunst 1998–2015.* Textband. Mattes, Heidelberg.

Evertz K (2021) "The prenatal dimension: Images in art and therapy". In: Evertz K et al. (eds.) *Handbook for prenatal psychology – Integrating research and practice.* Springer, Heidelberg, New York, 713–751.

Evertz K (2022) "Die Welt neu spüren – Die transgenerational-systemisch und pränatal fundierte methodenintegrative Psychotherapie – Integrative Kunst- und Körpertherapie." In: Klippel-Heidekrüger M, Janus L (eds.) *Vielfältige Zugänge zum vorsprachlichen und geburtlichen Erleben.* Mattes, Heidelberg, S. 271–292.

Evertz K, Janus L, Linder R (2014) *Lehrbuch der Pränatalen Psychologie.* Mattes, Heidelberg.

Evertz K, Janus L, Linder R (2021) *Handbook of prenatal and perinatal psychology.* Springer Nature, Cham, New York, Vandenhoeck & Ruprecht, Göttingen.

Gallagher S (2005) *How the body shapes the mind.* Oxford University Press, New York.

Gallese V (2013) *Den Körper im Gehirn finden - Konzeptuelle Überlegungen zu den Spiegelneuronen.* https://doi.org/10.13109/9783666451300.75

Gallese V (2023) *Von vorgeburtlichen Beziehungen zur Konstitution des Selbst*. Eine Neurobehaviorale Perspektive auf den primären Narzissmus. Vortrag, Sandler-Symposium, Wien, unveröffentlicht.

Gluckman P, Hanson M (2004) *The fetal matrix. Evolution, development and disease*. Cambridge University Press, New York.

Gluckman P, Hanson M (2006) *Developmental origins of health and disease*. Cambridge University Press, New York.

Harms T (2017) *Auf die Welt gekommen: Die neuen Baby-Therapien* (Neue Wege für Eltern und Kind). Psychosozial, Gießen.

House S (1999) "Primal integration therapy -School of Lake". In: *International Journal of Prenatal and Perinatal Psychology and Medicine* 11(4): 437–457.

Janus L (2000) *Die Psychoanalyse der vorgeburtlichen Lebenszeit und der Geburt*. Psychosozial, Gießen.

Janus L (2014) "Die Geschichte der Pränatalen Psychologie". In: Evertz K et al. (eds.) *Lehrbuch der Pränatalen Psychologie*. Mattes, Heidelberg, 3–11.

Janus L (2016) *Menschheitsgeschichte als psychologischer Entwicklungsprozess*. Mattes, Heidelberg.

Janus L (2020) *Unfertig – Werdend – Kreativ*. Mattes, Heidelberg.

Janus L (2021) The history of prenatal psychology. In: Evertz K et al. (eds.) *Handbook of prenatal psychology*. Springer, New York, 3–8.

Janus L (2024) *Revision der Freudschen Triebtheorie*. Unveröffentlicht.

Janus L, Evertz K (2008*) Kunst als kulturelles Bewusstsein geburtlicher und vorgeburtlicher Erfahrungen*. Mattes, Heidelberg.

Klippel-Heidekrüger M, Janus L (2022) *Vielfältige Zugänge zum vorsprachlichen und geburtlichen Erleben*. Mattes, Heidelberg.

Lewin K (1963/2012) *Feldtheorie in den Sozialwissenschaften*. Huber, Bern.

Metz G, Hoover T (2021) "Transgenerational consequences of perinatal experiences: programming of health and disease from mother to child and subsequent generations". In: Evertz K et al. (eds.) *Handbook for prenatal psychology – Integrating research and practice*. Springer, Heidelberg, New York, 63–81.

Ott M, Singer M, Hannemann J, Bliem HR, Schubert C (2016) "Wird mit onkologischen Erkrankungen vor dem Hintergrund psychoneuroimmunologischer Erkenntnisse aktuell angemessen umgegangen?" In: *Deutsche Zeitschrift für Onkologie* 48: 144–151.

Ott M, Singer M, Bliem HR, Schubert C (2021) "Prenatal psychoneuroimmunology" In: Evertz K et al. (eds.) *Handbook of prenatal and perinatal psychology*. Springer Nature, Cham, 115–147.

Parncutt R (2009) "Prenatal development and the phylogeny and ontogeny of musical behavior". In: Hallam S, Cross I, Thaut M (eds.) *Oxford handbook of music psychology*. Oxford Uni- versity Press, Oxford, 219–228.

Pert C (1998) *Molecules of Emotions*. Simon and Schuster, London.

Plagemann A (2011) *Perinatal programming – The state of the art*. De Gruyter, Berlin, New York.

Raffai J (2014) "Auswirkungen von Elternkonflikten im intrauterinen Raum". In: Evertz K et al. (eds.) *Lehrbuch der Pränatalen Psychologie*. Mattes, Heidelberg, 556–570.

Rank O (1927) Grundzüge einer genetischen Psychologie I und II. Deuticke Leipzig, Wien.

Rank O (1929) Technik der Psychoanalyse, Band II. Deuticke Leipzig, Wien.

Rank O (1931) Technik der Psychoanalyse, Band III. Deuticke Leipzig, Wien.

Sloterdijk P (1998ff) Sphären 1-3. Suhrkamp, Stuttgart.

Schwab M (2009) "Intrauterine Programmierung von Störungen der Hirnfunktion im späteren Leben". In: *Gynäkol Geburtshilfliche Rundsch* 49: 13–28.

Van den Bergh BR (2014) "Antenatal anxiety and stress and the neurobehavioural development of the fetus and child: Links and possible mechanisms". In: Evertz K, Janus L, Linder R (eds.) *Lehrbuch der Pränatalen Psychologie.* Mattes, Heidelberg, 70–103.

Van den Bergh BR, van den Heuvel MI, Lahti M, Braeken M, de Rooij SR, Entringer S, Schwab M (2017) "Prenatal developmental origins of behavior and mental health: The influence of maternal stress in pregnancy". In: *Neuroscience & Behavioral Reviews* 117: 26–64.

Van den Bergh BR, (2021) "Prenatal developmental origins of early brain and behavior development, of self-regulation in adolescence, and of cognition and central and autonomic nervous system function in adulthood". In: Evertz K et al. (eds.) *Handbook for prenatal psychology – Integrating research and practice.* Springer, Heidelberg, New York, 83–114.

Verdult R (2014) "Pränatale Bindungsentwicklung – auf dem Weg zu einer pränatalen Entwicklungspsychologie". In: Evertz K, Janus L, Linder R (eds.) Lehrbuch der Pränatalen Psychologie. Mattes, Heidelberg, 205–231.

Verdult R (2021) "Prenatal roots of attachment". In: Evertz K et al. (eds.) *Handbook of prenatal and perinatal psychology.* Springer Nature, Cham, New York, 227–246.

Verny T (2021) *The embodied mind. Understanding the mysteries of cellular memory, consciousness and our bodies.* Pegasus Books, New York, London.

Yehuda R, Lehrner A (2018) "Intergenerational transmission of trauma effects: Putative role of epigenetic mechanism". In: *World Psychiatry* 17(3): 243–257.

5

CHRONOLOGICAL CLASSIFICATION OF PRENATAL PSYCHOLOGY

This chapter describes a chronological order of prenatal psychology (PP). PP as a bio-psycho-social model assumes that all factors that affect a new child are important from the very beginning. This requires an overview of the following conditions:

1 Evolutionary conditions
2 Cultural, political and social conditions
3 Transgenerational and family system conditions
4 The history, constitution and emotional state of the parents
5 The comprehensive circumstances before and during conception: the bonding and relationship qualities of the parents' love
6 All bio-psycho-social influencing factors during pregnancy
7 All bio-psycho-social influencing factors before, during and after birth and within the first months of life

PP assumes that the wealth of factors involved in conception and pregnancy can be understood not only biologically but also in terms of attachment and relationship theory. In deeply regressive art and body psychotherapy and psychotherapeutic settings, we can also understand many aspects periconceptually and prenatally and not just postnatally.

PP is essentially concerned with the possibilities of the realities of pregnancy and birth for mother, child and father. The therapist Helga Fink speaks of a "womb–mother–father space" when self-awareness groups go into regressive processes in order to allow the prenatal history of each participant to become tangible. This term is intended to show that every pregnancy is one big story of three people. From the point of view of PP, everything that is successful and

DOI: 10.4324/9781003480242-5

everything that is problematic in a pregnancy is always an expression of the bonding and relationship qualities of the triangulation between father, mother and child. From the point of view of PP, there are therefore no exclusively biological conditions for particular events in a pregnancy but always bio-psycho-social conditions. The question is rather which resources medicine and psychology develop together to answer and treat pregnancy complications. There is no question that sometimes biological-medical strategies take priority, but sometimes psychological-emotional strategies are also needed. The point here is that PP is about the overdue integration of psychosomatic and psychotherapeutic and psychoneuroimmunological knowledge into prenatal biology and medicine, which is still underrepresented in the care of pregnant women and their intrauterine children.

1 Transgenerationality – preconception dynamics
2 Periconceptual psychology – conception dynamics
3 Prenatal psychology – prenatal dynamics
4 Perinatal psychology – birth dynamics, birth intervention dynamics
5 Early postnatal conditions – postpartum dynamics

These five temporal phases of PP are the five fundamental fields of prenatal medical and psychological research. In psychotherapy, these five fields should already be clarified in the anamnesis!

These five phases are psychologically significant for mother, father and child in various forms. Here it is decided which primal unhappiness (primal pain) and which primal happiness determine a person's life.

It is important and significant, especially in psychotherapies and psychosocial support during pregnancy, that all factors of all five phases are kept in view as far as possible. For example, from a medical and psychosomatic point of view, the aetiology of pre-eclampsia at the end of a pregnancy naturally has to do with the conditions of the first and second phases, especially with the factors of implantation, which in turn has to do with the history of the mother and father.

The following list provides a brief overview of biological prenatal development:

1 Conception: Fertilisation of the egg by a sperm leads to the formation of a fertilised egg, which implants in the uterus.
2 First trimester (weeks 1–12): During this phase, the embryo's organs develop and the placenta forms. The expectant mother may struggle with nausea, tiredness and mood swings.
3 Second trimester (weeks 13–27): The foetus grows rapidly and begins to move. The expectant mother may experience an increase in abdominal girth and noticeable foetal movements.

4 Third trimester (weeks 28–40): The foetus continues to gain weight and the organs continue to mature. The expectant mother may experience complaints such as back pain, water retention and sleep problems.
5 Birth: Labour begins and the baby is born. This marks the end of the pregnancy phase and the beginning of parenthood.

An initial overview of prenatal development as bio-psycho-social development

Prenatal developmental psychology is concerned with the development of the foetus and its developing brain, as well as its initial but basic emotional bonding experiences and abilities during pregnancy. Here are some important aspects that are studied in this field:

1 Prenatal development: This covers the various stages of foetal development, from fertilisation to birth. Various aspects such as the growth of organs and tissues, the formation of the nervous system and the development of sensory organs are analysed.
2 Influence of the environment: Prenatal development is strongly influenced by the environment in which the foetus finds itself. Factors such as nutrition, stress, drug use, smoking and alcohol consumption can have an impact on development.
3 Prenatal bonding: a form of bonding between the child and the parents arises at conception and develops prenatally until birth. The mother is the first experience of the world and her constitution determines how the world is experienced.
4 Studies have shown that stimuli such as the mother's voice or touching the abdomen can have an effect on the foetus's behaviour.
5 Early sensory experiences: The foetus is able to perceive and respond to sensory stimuli. Studies have shown that it can react to sounds, light and touch.
6 Prenatal learning: There is evidence that the foetus can already learn in the womb. For example, they can recognise certain sounds and react to repeated stimuli.
7 Effects on later development: Prenatal development can have an impact on the child's later cognitive, emotional and behavioural development. Studies have shown that certain prenatal factors can increase the risk of developmental disorders or behavioural problems.
8 Prenatal intervention: In some cases, prenatal interventions can be carried out to support the development of the foetus or to treat potential problems. This can include, for example, medical treatment or a change in diet, but especially psychological support for the parents, such as attachment analysis and emotional parenting programmes.

It is important to note that prenatal developmental psychology is a complex field of research that has not yet found an institutional framework, partly because it is genuinely transdisciplinary and this has overstretched the existing organisation of science and it has therefore not found an adequate place. However, the above-mentioned aspects provide an initial overview of some of the most important topics being investigated in this field.

Transgenerationality – preconception dynamics

Transgenerationality refers to the transfer of traits, behaviours or experiences from one generation to the next (Figure 5.1). Here are some of the most important factors that can contribute to transgenerationality:

1 Genetics: Genetic inheritance plays a role in the transmission of certain characteristics and traits from parents to their children. This includes physical and psychological characteristics such as eye colour, height and hair colour but also bio-psycho-social factors, potentials and talents, as well as genetically determined diseases or susceptibilities.
2 Family culture and values: Families often have certain cultural norms, values and traditions that are passed on from one generation to the next. These can influence the behaviour, attitudes and lifestyle of family members.

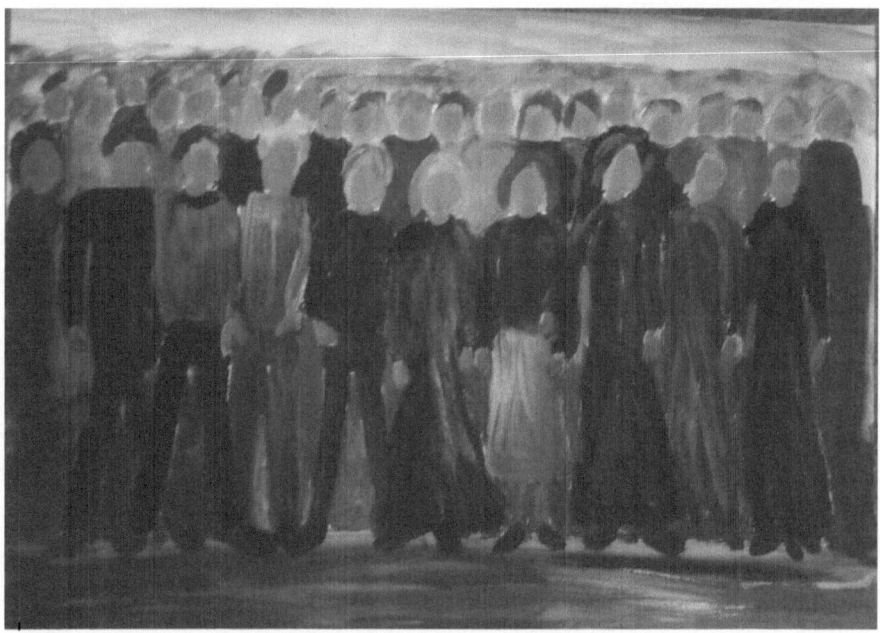

FIGURE 5.1   The ancestors – an art-therapeutic image of the ancestors.

3 Parenting patterns: The way in which parents raise their children can have an impact on their behaviour and attitudes. Certain parenting patterns or styles can be passed down through generations and shape the behaviour of offspring.
4 Traumatic experiences: Traumatic events or experiences in a family can have an impact on subsequent generations. This is sometimes referred to as transgenerational traumatisation and can lead to emotional or psychological stress.
5 Family role patterns: In many families, there are certain role patterns or dynamics that are passed on from one generation to the next. For example, traditional gender roles or family hierarchies can persist across generations.
6 Communication patterns: The way in which families communicate with each other can have an impact on subsequent generations. Communication patterns such as conflict avoidance, aggression or passivity can be passed on across generations.
7 Family resources and burdens: The availability of resources such as education, financial stability or social support in a family can have an impact on subsequent generations. Family stresses such as poverty, unemployment or family conflicts can also have transgenerational effects.

It is important to note that this list only covers some of the many factors of transgenerationality. The transfer of traits and experiences between generations is a complex process that is influenced by various individual, familial and societal factors.

Firstly, it should be clear that every person can only psychologically process, mourn and learn to integrate the traumas and conflict levels of their own existence since conception. However, the genetic information from the father and mother (and their ancestors) transports already resolved and unresolved traumas and levels of conflict. The biological and psychological transmission of this transgenerational life information is now well-researched (Elbert et al. 2006; Mansuy et al. 2014; Hoover & Metz 2021; Yao 2014).

Periconceptual psychology – conception dynamics

Patients in psychotherapeutic settings often express thoughts, fantasies and ideas about the connections between their physical or mental illness and early life events and pregnancy or birth complications but also with their conception. In addition to the positive sentences (Figure 5.2):

"I was a wanted child"
"My parents have been looking forward to seeing me for a long time"
"Her most fervent wish came true with me"

FERTILIZATION

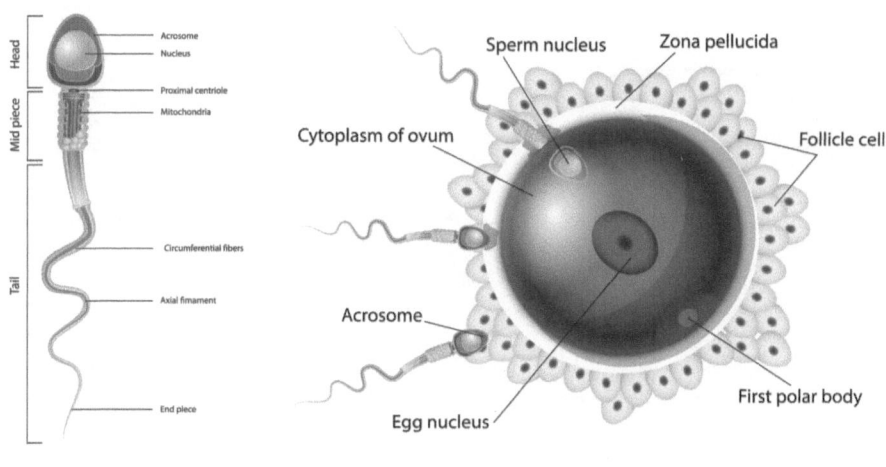

Spermatozoon   **Ovum**

FIGURE 5.2   Fertilisation.

Also include sentences like:

"My parents shouldn't have had any children."
"I don't know what they were thinking."
"I was not a love child. My parents were unhappy with each other."
"My conception was a rape."
"If I had been asked, I would have said no."
"I am an incest child. My real father was my grandfather."
"I come from an artificial insemination. I don't know who my father is."
"I only came about by chance."
"I wasn't wanted."
"My father was only there when I was conceived."

In addition to the concept of birth trauma, there is also the concept of procreative trauma in PP. People actually have a feeling for their origin and for the circumstances of their conception.

Or they express these contents symbolically in art-psychotherapeutic settings in symbolic forms and aesthetic dynamics, in body-psychotherapeutic settings in bodily sensations of diverse references to their life history, which are often also direct or indirect references to the deepest aetiologies up to the circumstances of conception (Evertz 2014, 2016, 2022).

In art therapy, positive conceptual memories are, for example, symbols of a bright origin, a sun, a star, a volcano, fireworks. More negative connotations

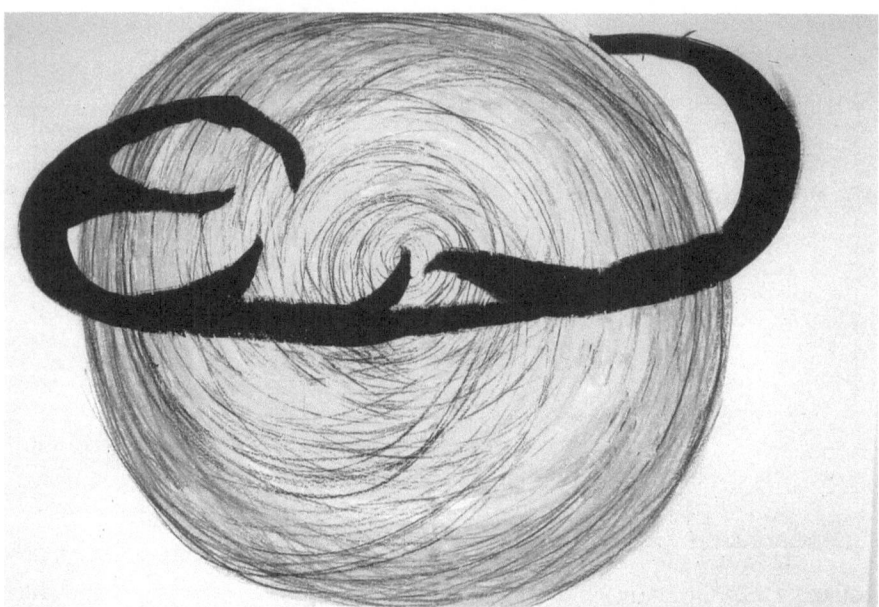

FIGURE 5.3 Conception Trauma

are very dark and deep abysses and tunnels. One adult patient painted her conception as a sun pierced by a black arrow: she was an incest child from her mother's union with her father, i.e. the client's grandfather.

A patient with the same conception trauma painted a sun with a black crown of thorns (see illustration) (Figures 5.3 and 5.4).

Positive support for young couples who want to become parents

Young, healthy parents are usually ready to embark on a marvellous process of transformation that can begin with the conscious conception of a child and indeed begins even before that. Long before conception, the couple already have inner images, ideas and fantasies of starting a family. Martin Dornes, a well-known infant researcher, once said: "Our life actually begins in the play of our parents, when mum and dad were still small children themselves and began to play family in the sandpit."

Topics for young parents before the conception of a child

– Are there intergenerational dynamics that are important to us?
– Can we accept trauma-informed, resilience- and healing-centred information and education?

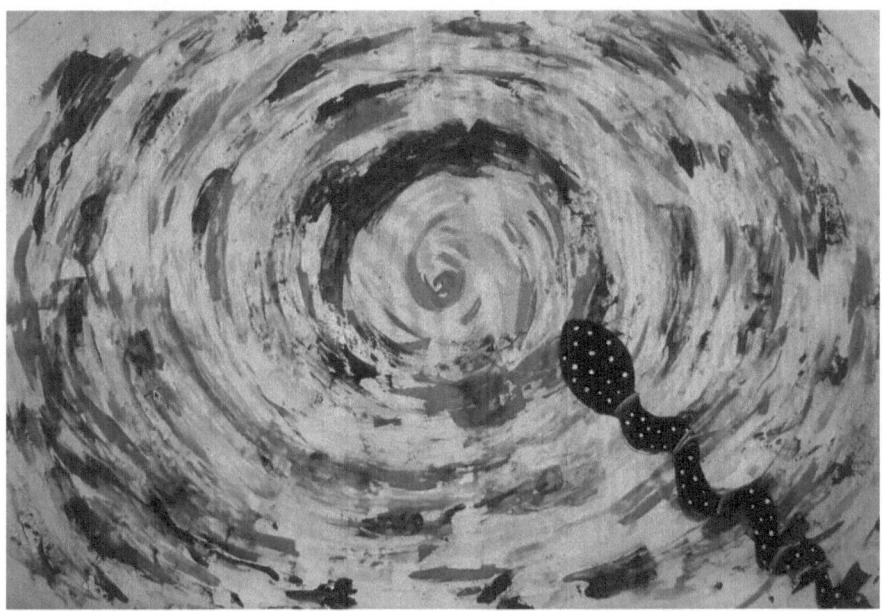

FIGURE 5.4 The following image shows a contaminated conception of a cancer patient as the penetration of a black sperm. The black sperm or the fear of the black infection. Paternal traumas as "life-negating messages" or maternal traumas, e.g. resulting in the rejection of one's own femininity, can show up in such images. This picture is about the systemic trauma that in three generations the fathers left their wives during pregnancy.

- Is there an awareness of the experiences of happiness, resilience and talents in our family systems?
- Are there and were there trauma-sensitive approaches and mourning skills for unfortunate experiences in our family systems?
- Can we create a welcoming space for a child?
- Do we want a conscious conception?
- Can we organise this as a party and celebration in our intimacy?
- Our baby should have the feeling that it is wanted and that everything is perfectly prepared.
- Don't we have to be too perfect and can we also be gracious towards our weaknesses?

According to WHO estimates, 41 per cent of pregnancies worldwide are unintended (WHO 2012). A recent study (BZgA 2016) from Germany found that around a third (33.7 per cent) of pregnancies were unintended (unintended/ambiguous/intended, but later). Almost 18 per cent of these

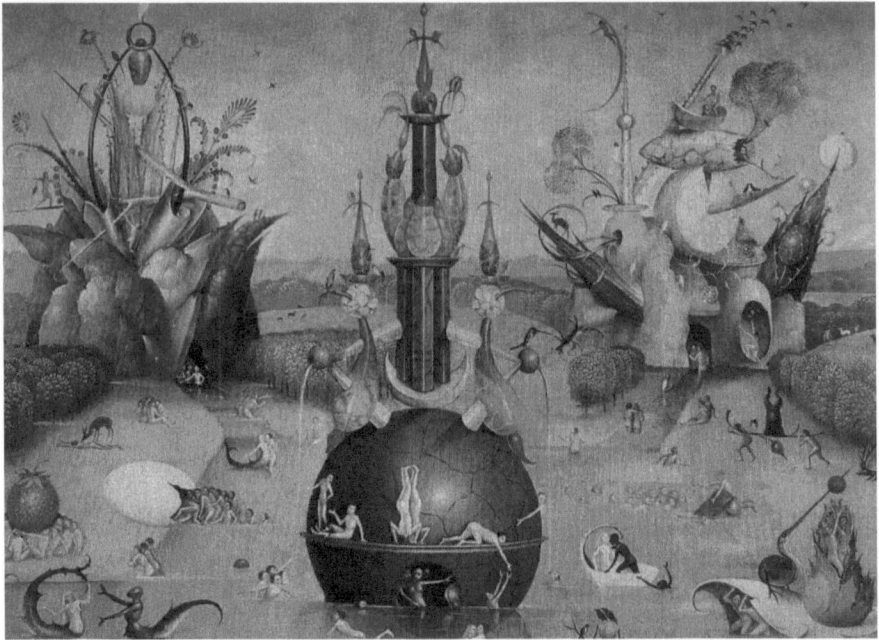

FIGURE 5.5 The excerpt from the triptych *The Garden of Earthly Delights* by Hieronymus Bosch (ca. 1490–1500) symbolises the immense complexity of conception. Paternal and maternal genetic material flow into a new egg, creating the new world of a new human being.

pregnancies were explicitly unintended, but more than half of them (57 per cent) were carried to term.

(Pro Familia 2016)

The problems arising from accidental or unwanted pregnancies can become very serious, so education should be provided not only on the biology but also on the psychology of parenthood. These topics should also be included in school education so that the culture of welcoming children becomes more loving and conscious (Figure 5.5).

The conditions for a healthy conception

The conditions for a healthy conception, i.e. the conception of a child, include various aspects. Here are some important conditions:

1 Physical health: Good physical health is important for a healthy conception. This includes a balanced diet, regular exercise, sufficient sleep and abstaining from harmful substances such as alcohol and tobacco.

2 Fertility: Sufficient fertility is required in both men and women to enable successful conception. This can be ensured by regular menstrual cycles in women and a sufficient number and quality of sperm in men.
3 Timing of intercourse: The likelihood of conception is highest when intercourse takes place during the fertile window. This is usually around the time of ovulation, when an egg is released and can be fertilised.
4 Absence of sexually transmitted infections (STIs): STIs can affect fertility and increase the risk of complications during pregnancy. It is important to get tested for STIs before conception and receive treatment if necessary.
5 Mental health: Good mental health can help to reduce stress and promote general well-being, which can have a positive impact on conception. It is important to manage stress and seek support for mental health issues to promote healthy conception.
6 Presence of a supportive environment: A supportive environment, whether in the form of a partner, family or friends, can help reduce stress and promote emotional well-being during the conception process.

It is important to note that the conditions for healthy conception can vary from couple to couple. If you are having difficulty getting pregnant or have questions about conception, you should consult a doctor or reproductive health professional.

Conception – implantation – discovery

These three events are formative relationship events for every person's life and are very fundamental to their ability to love and relate.

– What are the relationship qualities in the concept?
– What are the qualities of the relationship during implantation?
– What does the mother feel at the moment when she consciously realises that she is pregnant?

Conception

How are father and mother doing? How conscious are they of their desire to become parents? What ambivalences and fears, what pleasure and joy are there? It is actually about the big bang of every human existence in all its marvellous grandeur!

The two genetic gifts of the parents must be united by the child without contradiction. This terrible burden (and this marvellous gift (Evertz)) is imposed on each of us. At conception, the child is thrown into the web of relationships of the parents' partnership with all its lust, greed, grief, fear, excitement and ecstasy. In terms of its dowry, the child is just as identified with the father as it is with the mother. It can only establish an object relationship with the child via the internalised father. If this does not happen, the child must remain in this burying state that drills into the mother. It becomes indissolubly dependent on her.

(Meistermann-Seeger 1991)

Karlton Terry categorises the conception phase into 12 stages and assigns psychological themes to them:

12 STAGES OF HUMAN CONCEPTION

	Stage physiology	*Themes*
1	Sperm reaches cumulus oophorous	First contact salutations
2	Sperm blocked by corona radiata	Obstacles – defences
3	Decapitation – acrosome reaction zona	Losing our head
4	Hyperactivation – penetration	Entrapment embodiment
5	Perivitelline space – Penetration of the sperm head by vitelline fingers like Crown of thorns stabbings	Swimming – crocodile in the moat
6	Membrane fusion cortical granule	Destiny, delivery of centriole ejection of polar body
7	Pronuclear envelopes	Encapsulation – dance – attraction
8	Interdigitation	Break down of nucleus – intimate merging
9	Syngamy	Chaos and formlessness
10	Metaphase line-up	Structure 7 breakdown
11	Crossover and whirlwind	Mutation/destiny
12	First cell division	Architecture fixed

The psychological correlations result from observations of strong affects in deep regressive body-psychotherapeutic settings, the Sperm Journeys and Egg Journeys, and are richly documented (Figure 5.6) (Terry 2002).

Implantation

After conception and the journey in the fallopian tube, during which the fertilised egg is moved by a milky fluid, it falls into the uterus: a 64-cell ball that can no longer feed on its own (cor-starvation), hatches from the egg membrane (first birth) and seeks a place on the uterine lining.

It can only continue to live and develop if it has access to a source of nourishment - the mother's bloodstream. Her constitution and her mental and spiritual state are reflected in her mother's blood, as is her own history, beginning with the growth of her fertilised egg in her mother's body, in

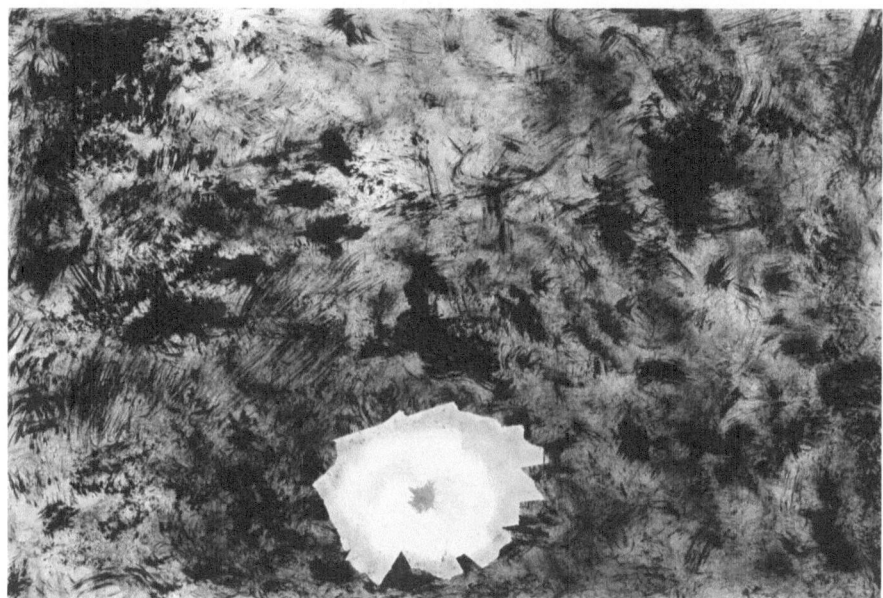

FIGURE 5.6   Painting of a cancer patient about her conception.

which the egg from which her child was then formed was already formed when the ovaries were laid in the growing embryo. The epigenetic imprinting by the maternal line of ancestors is sensed here in its full dimension!

The hungry cluster of cells, which eagerly wants to continue growing, can only do so by making contact and penetrating the uterine lining. The mother has to open herself up to a foreign being-to-be - created in an act of procreation between mother, father and the third party. At this point, 50–70% of the fertilised eggs are lost because there is not enough will to live? Because the female body closes up? Because not enough nourishment can be found? If there is enough for life to continue, an intensive metabolic exchange takes place between the great creaturely will to live of the cell cluster and the mother's personality, which has grown up through many imprints ("mother-fetal-cross-talk"). Cells also have memory and what is exchanged, what is negotiated?

(Fink 2022)

Discovery

How does the mother perceive the fact that she is really pregnant? From great joy and pleasure to terror and panic, all feelings can arise and are also perceived by the child (Table 5.1).

TABLE 5.1 Developmental Crises in the Primary Phase of Life

Sensitive or critical phase	Binding motif	Development crisis
Concept	First encounter	Primal trust ⇔ Primal inhibition/primal fear
Implantation	First connection	Living ⇔ Dying
Discovery	First realisation	Being wanted ⇔ Being unwanted
Umbilical affect (umbilical cord sensations)	First exchange	Promotion ⇔ Deprivation or intoxication
Birth	First transition/separation	Progress ⇔ Stagnation
Coining moment	First eye contact	Confirmation ⇔ Isolation
Psychological birth	First separation and individuality	Exploration ⇔ Fear of the unknown

Verdult (2014, p. 208).

Prenatal psychology – prenatal dynamics

Not only medically but also psychologically, it makes sense to categorise pregnancy into three trimesters.

– First trimester
– Second trimester
– Third trimester

We all know and generally expect wonderful images and feelings from pregnancy. Pregnancy should be ideal and beautiful. But there is no such thing as an ideal pregnancy. There is a wide spectrum of feelings, of pregnancy ambivalence, from rather affirmative to rather negative feelings. As a rule, mixtures determine the emotional state of expectant mothers, which can also change considerably during these three trimesters. As a rule, however, the feelings of mothers are relatively constant if no extraordinary events influence the pregnancy. The passing on of life is always associated with joy and hope as well as fears, questions and doubts. However, there are always unconscious images of the difficulties and threats and real traumas of and in pregnancies in the transgenerational family memory.

During pregnancy, this general problem of psychological entanglement and the risk of confusion become directly very significant and also physically very concrete. Never before are two people so intensely connected physiologically and therefore also psychologically as during these nine months. And never before are the positive and also the ambivalent and negative feelings or even traumatically generated non-feelings so tangible and effective and also manifest themselves in later life and can be felt and remembered in real terms (Evertz 2020, 2022).

The pregnant woman therefore actually integrates at least three "foreign levels" and establishes an immune tolerance at implantation and during pregnancy between:

1 The man's stranger (and his family history)
2 One's own split-off "stranger" (unresolved introjects from one's own history, which always tend to be life-negating) and
3 The strangeness of the child's uniqueness, beginning at conception, as a unique mixture of father and mother at this point in time, and as a "strange" new third living being with its own history beginning at conception!

The most important intrauterine process from an attachment-analytic perspective is the biological development of growing out of the mother's womb and the psychological development from the boundlessness, unity and sameness of maternal and foetal experiences, from the mother's psychological realm to a differentiated self/ego (Raffai 2014, p. 556).

The pregnant woman is more likely to react to all these challenges with physical symptoms if too much anxiety and depression are unresolved. Bleeding, premature contractions, retarded foetuses, prematurely ageing placenta, placenta previa, serial abortions, HELLP syndrome, intrauterine death, infertility, artificial insemination, etc. are ultimately physical/emotional emergency solutions resulting from an often unrecognised inner stress.

Psychodiagnostically, we often find the following in these symptoms: dependency conflicts with the parents, psychological immaturity, pre- and perinatal trauma in the family system, severe psychosocial stress factors during pregnancy, etc. (Raffai 2014, p. 557; Evertz 2020, 2021a).

Extreme pregnancy ambivalence manifests itself in abortion, abortion attempts or abortion fantasies:

• Unconscious motive: to escape the threat of annihilation by merging with the object
• Unconscious dynamics: re-enactment of own early traumatisation – longing for control over death
• Unconscious hope: to break the cycle through abortion, to get rid of the "inner fear child" (Meistermann 1991; Evertz 2021a).

The most common psychodynamic in the pregnancy conflict is therefore the confusion between the "inner" traumatised child (i.e. the early childhood, pre- and perinatal psychological part of the history of the father and mother (and their family history)) and the real child growing up in the uterus (Evertz 2020, 2021).

Bodywork (Emerson 2021; Marlock & Weiss 2006; Terry 2014) and pictorial levels (Evertz 2002, 2017, 2021b) offer very good approaches to pre- and perinatal and early childhood trauma in adult and child therapy:

- Artistic-aesthetic
- Body psychotherapeutic
- Art psychotherapeutic
- Psychotherapeutic

Prenatal introjects are so fundamental to a biography that they have not yet become a general topic of therapy under concepts of fate and fantasies of destiny, i.e. religiously or otherwise repressed. They are so strongly declared in our emotional life as having "always been there" that many people do not succeed in clarifying and differentiating them from the actual "self" that still lies beneath, the "selfness" that Balint and Meistermann spoke of, or are only understood in the life crises of later life and addressed in a conflict-resolving manner.

In today's baby and paediatric therapies, however, it is clear that the earlier symptoms are also subjected to a thorough anamnesis of prenatal and birth conditions, the easier and faster it is to heal babies and children, which takes months and years in later adult therapies (Terry 2014; Renggli 2013).

In the psychotherapy of adults, too, deep connections between the current crisis situation and the beginning of life repeatedly emerge (Figure 5.7). A cancer patient says the following sentence during end-of-life counselling.

The patient saw two forms in the picture, like a mother cell and a child cell or like a mother cancer cell and a child cancer cell. The atmosphere is cold, the relationship unclear (18 × 24 cm).

I was able to work through this mother-daughter conflict with the patient to such an extent that she was able to accept dying and death in a much more relaxed and relieved way.

Perinatal psychology – birth dynamics, birth intervention dynamics

The birth of a child changes everything in a couple's life. Birth is one of the most important life events because it is an exemplary, condensed event of relationship and life dynamics and at the same time establishes a strong and conscious body experience. In a spontaneous birth, we practise how a good relationship can transition into a more mature form of relationship through a separation. How mother and child can experience how living together ends up being too dense and too heavy and would prevent future growth and development for both if a detachment does not take place. This detachment is set in motion by the child and now it is about how, in the best-case scenario, mother and child work together to bring the process to a successful

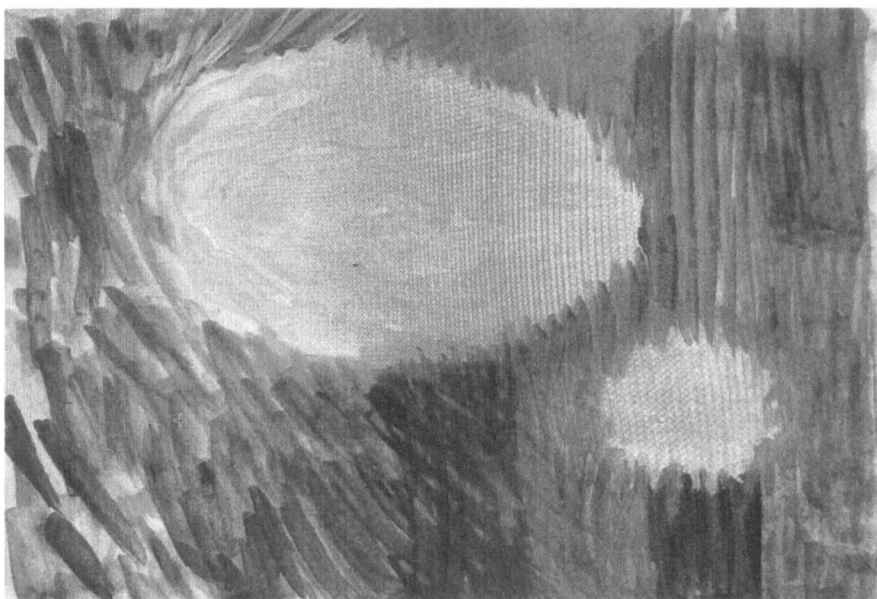

FIGURE 5.7 "My mother would rather have a tumour than be pregnant with me. Now she's won. Now I am the tumour". She painted this picture (DIN A4).

conclusion, with the aim of meeting again and for the first time at the same time. They have known each other for a long time but not yet as separate living beings. They know each other from the inside but only to a limited extent from the outside.

The birth process has a strong influence on body image and body schema. Experiencing one's own body as a strong force that is robust and full of energy in the face of a challenge activates a healthy self-perception as a physical, mental and spiritual being. Of course, this can only follow on from and build on a healthy, clear object relationship during pregnancy, where clear body boundaries have already been experienced.

In the birth process, great forces normally have to be set in motion or allowed to be set in motion. Instinctive patterns have to be recognised. Mothers unanimously report that at a certain point in labour, they had to give up a certain amount of control in order to make room for a greater force. Births become complicated when this is not possible, when mothers become too tense, withdraw into themselves and can no longer perceive the joint effort. The child then feels abandoned and often struggles alone without success. Nothing moves forward any more. Many patients later report a pattern of "it won't go forward and it won't go back" in the therapies, right through to an agonising feeling of having to go on to dissociation and, in the worst case, to a fear and panic of having to die now before the child falls into shock and no longer perceives anything. This means a split between self-perception and perception of others and has far-reaching consequences.

The successful process of a spontaneous birth forms the basis for a strong self-confidence to be able to set great things in motion and bring them to a good end. The entire hormonal system learns that it is worth making an effort and pushing yourself to the limit in order to "come through", to have conquered a new world, and to be rewarded with relaxation and new kinds of touch and security. And ultimately through a new kind of freedom and autonomy!

The complex biopsychological processes create a paradigm for all future threshold events in life and the possibilities of successfully coping with them (Janus Birth).

In the case of more complicated births, this training for life is made more difficult, to the point of fear of change altogether. Later transitions, tests, threshold events and special challenges are experienced more anxiously or avoided.

Good birth support is characterised by the following features:

1 Empathy and sensitivity: The accompanying person should be empathetic and respect the needs of the expectant mother.
2 Expertise: The accompanying person should have a sound knowledge of obstetrics and be able to convey medical information in an understandable way.
3 Support and encouragement: The carer should support, encourage and reassure the mother-to-be throughout the birth process.
4 Respect for the woman's autonomy: The accompanying person should respect the expectant mother's decisions and support her in acting independently.
5 Continuity and trust: Good labour support builds on a trusting relationship between the support person and the expectant mother and accompanies her continuously throughout the entire birth process.
6 Flexibility and adaptability: The accompanying person should be able to adapt to the individual needs and wishes of the expectant mother and react flexibly to changes in the birth process.
7 Calm and serenity: Good labour support radiates calm and serenity to calm and support the expectant mother in stressful situations.
8 Discretion and confidentiality: The accompanying person should handle personal information sensitively and ensure a confidential atmosphere.

Overall, good birth support is characterised by compassion, expertise, support, respect, trust and empathy.

Early postnatal conditions – postpartum dynamics

The miracle of birth should continue with comprehensive care and love for the child. The parents fall in love with their baby, the joy of parenthood. Many people count the birth of their children as one of the most important and profound experiences of their lives. The first contact, the first greeting, the first perception of the trinity, the first physical contact is called "the sacred hour". In fact, these first moments, days and weeks of a child's arrival are a time of special peace for many families. And indeed, the qualities of these first experiences of the born child mean a further fundamental strengthening of its identity and its basic trust.

But many women also experience childbirth as difficult and even traumatic. There is always a connection here to the quality of the prenatal relationship between mother and child.

> The quality of attachment has also been linked to the mother's perinatal mental health. Weak prenatal attachment has been associated with postpartum anxiety (Blumberg, 1980; Gaffney, 1989) and depression during pregnancy and the postpartum period (Brandon et al., 2007; Condon & Corkindale, 1997; Lindgren, 2001). On the other hand, in a sample of women in Israel, strong attachment was found to moderate susceptibility to postpartum depression (Priel & Besser, 1999). Factors of personal susceptibility to depression were measured, and highly self-critical women reported less depression if they had a strong attachment to the foetus during pregnancy.
>
> *(Brandon 2009, p. 216f)*

Recommendations for young parents

- Rhythm, warmth and consistency: The early relationship is the most important for your child's whole life. Provide security, warmth and love but don't overburden yourself.
- A romantic relationship is not a sure-fire success. Both your relationship as a couple and your relationship with your child are subject to constant change and require a willingness to learn and openness to new things.
- Your child sometimes demands a lot from you: Sleepless nights, the stress of experiencing your child's crying, anxiety in the event of illness, even if it is mild. Get support and make sure you have free time for mum, dad and child.
- A child wants strong parents! Grow with your child to greater personal maturity!
- Take turns looking after the child and involve other people as well.
- Talk openly about your feelings!
- A three-way relationship can mean different dyads. Sometimes there is a closer bond in one dyad, sometimes in the other. Just be lovingly jealous.

Many counselling institutions offer help and support for young parents:

> Who gets up at night? Who changes the next nappy? Who will put the baby to bed the next night? The birth of your child brings new tasks into your everyday life. It is therefore important that you discuss together as a couple how you want to tackle the new tasks and divide them up. If the division of tasks is not clear, conflicts can quickly arise - especially if one person in the relationship feels they have to do everything on their own. But even if the division of tasks works well for you, there can always be moments when you feel overwhelmed or simply run out of energy. It's not just you, but a lot of parents. Getting support and help is a sign of strength and nothing to be ashamed of.
>
> *(Caritas 2024)*

Summary

The chronological system of PP makes it easier to organise events and aetiologies in the fundamental basic conditions of an individual's life.

1 Transgenerationality – preconception dynamics
2 Periconceptual psychology – conception dynamics
3 Prenatal psychology – prenatal dynamics
4 Perinatal psychology – birth dynamics, birth intervention dynamics
5 Early postnatal conditions – postpartum dynamics

(see also Chapters 7–9)

Literature

Brandon A (2009) "History of the theory of prenatal attachment". In: *Journal of Prenatal and Perinatal Psychology Health* Summer; 23(4): 201–222.

Caritas (2024) "Beratungsangebote für junge Eltern". *Google*, April 2024.

Elbert T, Rockstroh B, Kolassa I, Schauer M, Neuner F (2006) "The influence of organized violence and terror on brain and mind – A co-constructive perspective". In: Baltes P, Reuter-Lorenz P, Rösler F (eds.) *Lifespan development and the brain: The perspective of biocultural co-constructivism*. Cambridge University Press, Cambridge, 326–349.

Emerson W (2014) "Prä- und Perinataler Schock". In: Evertz K, Janus L, Linder R (eds.) *Lehrbuch der Pränatalen Psychologie*. Mattes, Heidelberg, 520–546.

Emerson W (2021) "Psychotherapy with infants and children". In: Evertz K et al. (eds.) *Handbook for prenatal psychology – Integrating research and practice*. Springer Nature, Heidelberg, New York, 543–558.

Evertz K (2002) *Kunstanalyse*. Mattes, Heidelberg.

Evertz K (2014) *Lehrbuch der Pränatalen Psychologie*. Mattes, Heidelberg.

Evertz K (2016) "A visual exploration of psychodynamics in problematic pregnancies: Case studies in analytic-aesthetic art therapy". In: *Journal of Prenatal and Perinatal Psychology and Health* 31(2): 107–133.

Evertz K (2017) *Das Erste Bild – Pränatale Ästhetik. Schriften zur Kunst 1998–2015.* Textband. Mattes, Heidelberg.

Evertz K (2020) "The inner child or the "inner child"? Confusion during pregnancy and its lifelong consequences". In: Gouni O et al. (eds.) *Change - Birthing & parenting at times of crisis.* Cosmoanelixis, Athens, 2021, S. 293–334.

Evertz K (2021a) "A visual exploration of psychodynamics in problematic pregnancies: Case studies in analytic-Aesthetic art therapy". In: Evertz K et al. (eds.) *Handbook for prenatal psychology – Integrating research and practice.* Springer, Heidelberg, New York, 309–331.

Evertz K (2021b) "The prenatal dimension: Images in art and therapy". In: Evertz K et al. (eds.) *Handbook for prenatal psychology – Integrating research and practice.* Springer Nature, Cham, New York, 713–751.

Evertz K (2022) "Die Welt neu spüren – Die transgenerational-systemisch und pränatal fundierte methodenintegrative Psychotherapie – Integrative Kunst- und Körpertherapie". In: Klippel-Heidekrüger M, Janus L (eds.) *Vielfältige Zugänge zum vorsprachlichen und geburtlichen Erleben.* Mattes, Heidelberg, S. 271–292.

Evertz K, Janus L, Linder R (2021) *Handbook of prenatal and perinatal psychology.* Springer Nature, Cham, New York.

Fink H (2022) *Einnistung.* Workshop Flyer, unveröffentlicht.

Hoover T, Metz G (2021) "Transgenerational Consequences of perinatal experiences: programming of health and disease from mother to child and subsequent generations". In: Evertz K et al. (eds.) *Handbook of prenatal psychology.* Springer Nature, New York, 63–82.

Janus L (2015) *Geburt.* Psychosozial, Gießen.

Mansuy I, Gapp K, Jawaid A, Sarkies P, Bohacek J, Pelczar P, Prados J, Farinelli L, Miska E (2014) "Implication of sperm RNAs in transgenerational inheritance of the effects of early trauma in mice". *Nature Neuroscience* 17: 667–669. Doi: 10.1038/nn.3695, 2014.

Marlock G, Weiss H (2006) *Handbuch der Körperpsychotherapie.* Schattauer, Stuttgart.

Meistermann-Seeger E (1991) "Wodurch kommt es zur Abtreibung? – Diagnose einer psycho-biologischen Krise." Vortrag 25.6.1991, Erftstadt-Lechenich, Katholisches Bildungswerk im Erftkreis, unveröffentlicht.

Pro familia: BZgA Bundeszentrale für gesundheitliche Aufklärung (Hg.) (2016) *frauen leben 3. Familienplanung im Lebenslauf von Frauen.* Schwerpunkt: Ungewollte Schwangerschaften. Eine Studie im Auftrag der BZgA von Cornelia Helfferich, Heike Klindworth, Yvonne Heine, Ines Wlosnewski. Köln: BZgA. Online unter: publikationen.sexualaufkle rung.de/index.php?docid=4043 (Zugriff: 5.2.18).

Raffai J (2014) "Auswirkungen von Elternkonflikten im intrauterinen Raum". In: Evertz K et al. (eds.) *Lehrbuch der Pränatalen Psychologie.* Mattes, Heidelberg, 556–570.

Renggli F (2013) *Das goldene Tor zum Leben.* London, Arkana.

Terry K (2002) *The sperm journey, the egg journey.* www.edicolibri.com, Out of print

Terry K (2014) "Pre- and perinatal baby therapy". In: Evertz K, Janus L, Linder R (eds.) *Lehrbuch der Pränatalen Psychologie.* Mattes, Heidelberg, 425–436.

Verdult R (2014) "Pränatale Bindungsentwicklung – auf dem Weg zu einer pränatalen Entwicklungspsychologie". In: Evertz K, Janus L, Linder R (eds.) *Lehrbuch der Pränatalen Psychologie.* Mattes, Heidelberg, 205–231.

Yao Y (2014) "Ancestral exposure to stress epigenetically programs preterm birth risk and adverse maternal and newborn outcomes". In: *BMC Medicine,* Springer nature, Cham. https://doi.org/10.1186/s12916-014-0121-6

6

PRENATAL PERCEPTION AND SENSORY DEVELOPMENT

Early sensory experiences in the womb

The description of prenatal perception involves two levels. On the one hand, there is extrospective research; on the other hand, there is introspective research. On the one hand, there is measurement and observation; on the other hand, it is about empathy and memory and therapeutic regression. Both research approaches are important and complement each other in prenatal psychology. In recent years, this knowledge has been fundamentally expanded, and the competences of the embryo and foetus as relational beings have become much more prominent. The child is in contact with its environment from the very beginning and can perceive much more than previously thought.

Prenatal perception and sensory development: an overview

The prenatal period is a crucial time for the development of the child, including the development of the senses and the ability to perceive. In this chapter, we will provide an overview of prenatal perception and sensory development, including the different senses that develop during this time and the stimuli to which the foetus can respond in the womb.

Prenatal psychology assumes a continuum of perception from the first cell. From the very beginning, we are a living system that is involved in incredibly complex reciprocal processes with the respective biotope. The development of visual, auditory, somatosensory, motor, proprioceptive, vestibular and visceral sensory modalities is therefore an unfolding and development of the preceding exchange processes between the cell, blastocyst, embryo and uterus.

DOI: 10.4324/9781003480242-6

Even before that, there was a complex developmental history of the egg in the ovary and fallopian tube and of the sperm in the testicles and on its way to the fallopian tube.

This means that multisensory integration is not a process of the organism that can be produced retrospectively, but conversely, the multisensory ability of the organism is a further development of an already amodal and synaesthetic holistic perception from the first cell. Otherwise, growth beyond the first cell would not be possible.

The patriarchal-male view of early human embryonic development needs to be expanded to include a female-maternal view. A bottom-up approach is a fundamentally different understanding than a top-down one. The female research perspective is more integrative, synthetic and focused on relationships, while the male research perspective is more analytical, dissecting and often also dissociative. Heuristically, we need both perspectives of research, but we still need to learn to think them together more, as prenatal psychology does.

Prenatal development is an unfolding process from one cell to billions of cells, each from the "knowledge" and "perception" of the previous cell development. The blastocyst naturally communicates with the mucous membrane of the uterine wall in order to find a place for implantation. Communication here means not only a biological-chemical-physical exchange process, but also psychosocial exchange processes expressed in these models. Two-thirds of all pregnancies end at implantation, often unnoticed, because something does not fit together in the bio-psycho-social field of the couple and the family systems (see Chapters 5, 8 and 9).

So sensory development is about multisensory unfolding for a unified reason as the actual achievement of our prenatal and early postnatal development! It is not about a laborious multisensory merging! (Evertz 2008; Verny 2021)

Holistic instead of just cross-modality

Numerous recent studies have demonstrated the ability of human newborns to combine information from different sensory modalities, such as touch and vision or vision and hearing, to recognise a person or object (for a review see Lickliter & Bahrick, 2007). Two hours after birth, newborns look longer at their mother's face than at an unfamiliar face if their mother has previously spoken to them, allowing them to associate her face with the voice heard and learnt in utero (Coulon, Guellaï, & Streri, 2011). Similarly, after a period of habituation to a video of a woman speaking, newborns are more likely to look at this familiar face in a choice test when the sound of her voice is added to the image during the habituation phase (Coulon et al., 2011; Guellaï et al., 2011). In the first days of life, they are also able to recognise the congruence or incongruence between lip movements and a vowel sound. This is evidence of audiovisual connections (Coulon, Hemimou, & Streri, 2013). Newborns can also transmit tactile and visual information. Less than 72 hours after birth, they are able to visually recognise objects (prism or cylinder) that they previously held in their hand (Streri & Gentaz, 2004). Newborns habituated to either a visual or tactile object (either a smooth or a rough cylinder) explored the unfamiliar object longer than the one they were habituated to when both objects were presented in the other perceptual modality (tactile or visual) (Sann & Streri, 2007). Again, they are able to transfer information received via one perceptual modality to another.

(Andre 2017, p. 355f)

The observation of early behavioural patterns since the early 1970s and 1980s already showed very pronounced movements, which were increasingly perceived not only as purely physiological patterns split off by autism but also as active and reactive behaviours demanding exchange and resonance!

First appearance of foetal behaviour (deVries 1982; DiPietro 2008)

- Barely noticeable movement: seventh week
- Startled twitching: eight week
- Hiccups: ninth week
- Isolated arm and leg movements: ninth week
- Head rotation: ninth/tenth week
- Breathing movements: tenth week
- Hand–face contact: tenth week
- Routes: tenth week
- Body rotation: tenth week
- Yawning: 11th week
- Finger movement: 12th week
- Sucking and swallowing: 12th week
- Burrowing movements: 14th week
- Eye movements: 16th week

Maturation of the most important brain centres:

- Hypothalamus, amygdala and mammillary body: fifth/sixth week of pregnancy
- Nucleus accumbens, septum and most important limbic connections: sixth/seventh week of pregnancy
- Amygdalar nuclei clearly distinguishable: seventh to ninth week of pregnancy

The world of the intrauterine child is therefore much richer in sensory and therefore also bio-psycho-social terms than has long been assumed. André provides a good overview of the current scientific findings on the sensory development of the intrauterine child (André 2018).

Development of the senses: scientific knowledge

During the prenatal phase, various senses develop in the foetus. The sense of hearing is one of the first senses to develop, and studies have shown that the foetus can react to sounds from its environment from as early as the third trimester. The sense of touch also develops early, and touch can trigger a reaction in the foetus. The sense of taste develops through the amniotic fluid that is swallowed by the foetus, while the sense of smell is not yet fully developed.

Stimuli and perception in the womb

The foetus can perceive and react to various stimuli from its environment. These include sounds such as the mother's voice or music, touch from movements or pressure from outside and taste stimuli from the amniotic fluid. Studies have shown that the foetus can react to these stimuli with movements or changes in the heartbeat. It is also assumed that the foetus is able to distinguish between different stimuli and develop preferences for certain stimuli.

Influence of prenatal perception on development

Prenatal perception and sensory development have an influence on the child's later development. Experiences in the womb can influence the formation of neuronal connections and support the development of the brain. Positive stimulation and interaction with the environment can promote cognitive, emotional and social development. In addition, appropriate prenatal awareness can help to establish an early bond between mother and child.

Factors that influence prenatal perception

Various factors can influence prenatal perception. These include genetic factors, environmental stimuli such as noise or stress, the mother's behaviour during pregnancy as well as nutrition and lifestyle factors. It is important to note that negative influences such as high levels of stress or harmful substances can also have a negative impact on prenatal development.

Conclusion

Prenatal perception and sensory development play an important role in the early development of the foetus.

The foetus's ability to perceive and react to various stimuli lays the foundation for the later development of the senses and interaction with the environment.

The classic five senses:

Sense of hearing
Sense of touch
Sense of taste
Sense of smell
Sense of sight

1 **Sense of hearing:** From the 16th week of pregnancy, babies in the womb can perceive sounds, especially their mother's voice and heartbeat. From the 24th week of pregnancy, they are also able to hear external sounds such as music or conversations from outside.

Changes in body movements can be observed after continuous transmission of a pure tone of 500 Hz with increasing intensity (from 65 dB to 120 dB) through the maternal abdominal wall (Hepper & Shahidullah, 1994). Foetuses also respond to various external vibroacoustic, musical or speech stimuli by changing their sucking and heart rate (Kisilevsky et al, 2009; Kisilevsky, Pang, & Hains, 2000; Leader, Baillie, Martin, & Vermeulen, 1982; Petrikovsky, Schifrin, & Diana, 1993; Visser, Mulder, Wit, Mulder, & Prechtl 1989).

(André 2018, p. 354)

2 **Sense of touch:** From the seventh week of pregnancy, the nerve endings on the foetus' lips and in the mouth begin to develop, enabling the first touch stimuli. From the 20th week of pregnancy, the nerve endings are distributed over the entire body and the baby can feel touch from the outside.

Sensory skin receptors are present at least 7 weeks post conception (PC) and are connected to the spinal cord at 8 weeks PC. However, the connections between the spinal cord and the brain are not established until later and are not functional until 20 to 24 weeks PC (Anand & Hickey, 1987; Glover & Fisk, 1999; Hamon, 1996; Laquerrière, 2010)... In twin pregnancies, evoked movements (i.e. evoked movements (i.e. a movement of one foetus after touching the other foetus within seconds) have been recorded in twin pregnancies from 12 weeks of age PC, and their occurrence increases with age, illustrating the maturation of tactile perception. A few hand-head movements can already be observed at 10 weeks PC and their frequency increases rapidly (deVries, Visser, &

Prechtl, 1985). In parallel, thumb sucking is rarely observed before 15 weeks, but becomes more frequent thereafter (Hepper, Shahidullah, & White, 1991). Pressure on the maternal abdomen can also be perceived by the foetus (from 32 to 40 weeks PC), which reacts with simultaneous heart rate changes (Bradfield, 1961; Issel, 1983; Walker, Grimwade, & Wood, 1973).

(André 2018, p. 351)

3 **Sense of taste:** From the seventh week of pregnancy, the taste buds develop in the foetus's mouth so that it can already perceive different flavours in the womb, which are transmitted through the amniotic fluid.

The taste buds appear in the 7th week and are fully developed in the 14th to 15th week (Hersch & Ganchrow, 1980; Witt & Reutter, 1997), while the taste receptors, which are mainly located in the taste buds, appear in the 11th to 12th week and become functional between the 13th and 15th week. At this stage, the receptors could become functional, as they are already connected to the taste buds via nerve fibres.

(Witt & Reutter 1998)

In a pioneering study, it was found that foetuses can swallow as early as 12 weeks of PC (Pritchard, 1965), so their taste perception was assessed by changing the composition of the amniotic fluid and recording the subsequent changes in swallowing rates. The swallowing rate of 34-week-old PC infants increases after an injection of saccharin and decreases after an injection of lipiodol into the amniotic fluid (Liley 1972). Therefore, at least at 34 weeks PC, fetuses seem to be able to express taste preferences or at least adapt their behaviour to what they perceive in the amniotic fluid.

(André 2018, p. 353)

4 **Sense of smell:** Although the sense of smell is not fully developed until after birth, babies in the womb can already perceive certain odours from the 28th week of pregnancy, which are absorbed via the amniotic fluid.

The main olfactory system consists mainly of an epithelium composed of numerous hair cells that appear in the seventh week of life and mature in the eleventh week of life (Piatkina, 1982). The trigeminal system appears in the 4th week with the appearance of the trigeminal nerve. Finally, the vomeronasal fibres can already be distinguished from those of the main olfactory system in the 7th week of PC. The olfactory bulb appears at 6 weeks PC, and the first synapses between nasal fibres and cortex are functional at 7–8 weeks PC (Bossy, 1980; Piatkina, 1982). Although most elements of the olfactory system are already present at 8 weeks, some develop later, such as the nasal receptors at 28 weeks (Chuah & Zheng, 1987). Because of the amniotic fluid surrounding the foetus, responses related to olfactory abilities are difficult to separate from those related to gustative abilities at the foetal stage. Consequently, the first evidence of responses to odours comes from studies on premature infants tested with airborne odorants.

(André 2018, p. 353)

5 **Sense of sight:** The sense of sight is the last sense to develop and is only fully developed after birth. Nevertheless, babies in the womb can perceive light and shadow from the 26th week of pregnancy, as their eyes are already functional.

The central zone of the retina (consisting mainly of cones, which are involved in colour vision) is not as developed at birth as the peripheral zones (consisting mainly of rods, which are involved in achromatic vision; Abramov et al., 1982). These peripheral zones (parafovea and midperipheral retina), in which the photoreceptors develop from 26 weeks PC, are functional at birth (Hendrickson & Drucker, 1992). Neural connections develop slowly from 26 to 29 weeks PC and continue to develop up to 15 months after birth (Burkhalter, Bernardo, & Charles, 1993). Reports show that fetuses respond physiologically (increased heart rate) and behaviourally (body movements) to extrauterine light (amnioscopy, light stimulation) (Kiuchi, Nagata, Ikeno, & Terakawa, 2000; Peleg & Goldman, 1980; Smyth, 1965). According to Fulford et al (2003), foetuses of at least 36 weeks PC respond to a light source of constant intensity diffused through the maternal abdomen with increased activity in their frontal cortex.

(André 2018, p. 354f)

Stimuli are necessary for a child's brain development and the development of the sensory organs. Only in a lively environment with constant interaction can the child develop and be prepared for the environment and later the outside world. Children whose mothers had limited motor skills during pregnancy or even had to lie down for a long period of time, e.g. due to premature labour or illness, grow up in a more monotonous environment, with the likelihood of certain deficits.

Other deficits can of course also arise if the mother is physically healthy but is caught up in strong ambivalences towards the child, for example, or represses or denies the pregnancy and does not really make psychological contact with the child (Figures 6.1–6.3).

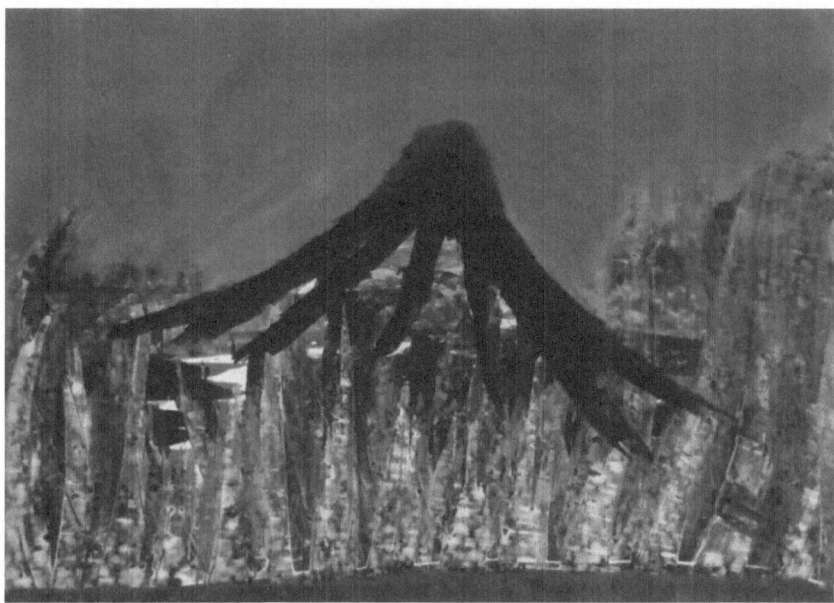

FIGURE 6.1 A 35-year-old female patient with a diagnosis of depression. Her mother fell ill during pregnancy and had to spend several months in hospital. An octopus-shaped shadow lies over a colourful abundance. The depression disappeared after the initiation of a mourning process over the "dead" during the pregnancy.

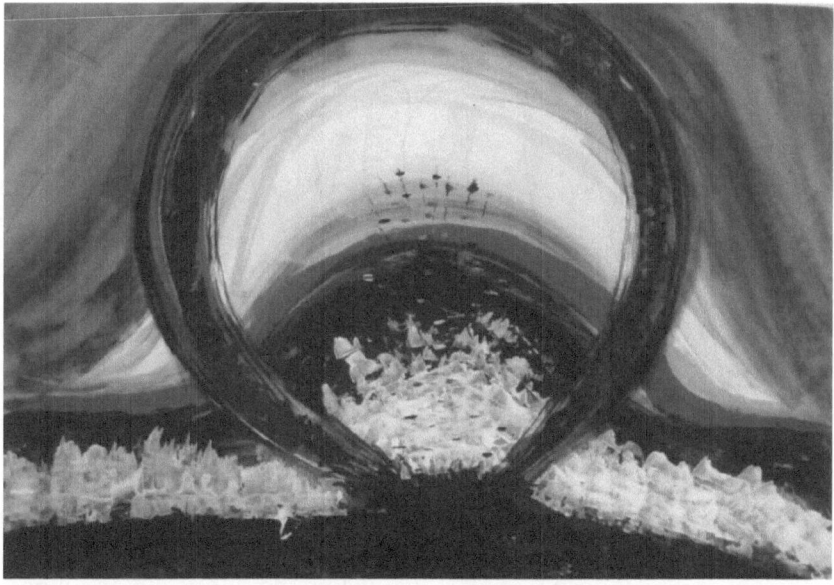

FIGURE 6.2 The same patient also deals with the complications of implantation.

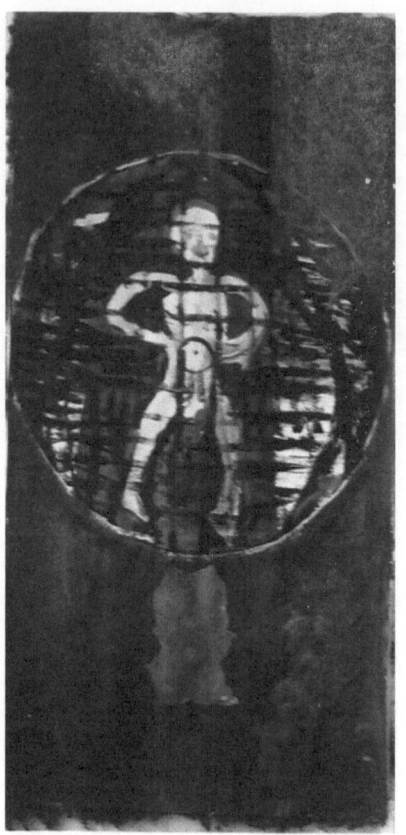

FIGURE 6.3 An artist expresses the intrauterine feeling of being at the mercy of the mother's depressive state, which is perceived as a prison.

In deep regressive body psychotherapy settings in which prenatal trauma can be re-experienced, many patients described extraordinarily exciting complex qualities of their own prenatal body experience and proprioceptive perception (Evertz 2022) (see also Chapter 9).

The rich sensory world of the intrauterine child

What does a baby experience in the womb and what does it feel? The bio-psycho-social research perspective asks about the real circumstances and the reality of the child's experience.

In addition to scientific research, prenatal psychology investigates the following conditions of intrauterine existence as experiential realities in an attachment and relationship context that determine our health and illnesses.

The prenatal space of experience creates fundamental patterns of perception of the world.

Prenatal patterns of perception

1 Being surrounded by something alive
2 Being dependent on something bigger
3 To be able to experience yourself as alive, the more the more resonances there are
4 A personal experience of growth
5 Levels of sensation for the development of your own physicality
6 A constant tapestry of sound. There is constant sound and movement, sometimes more, sometimes less (mother's voice, mother's heartbeat, blood flow in the blood vessels and organic sounds, external sounds, especially the father's voice and the mother's reaction to it). However, it is mainly low-frequency sounds below 100 Hz (60–90 dB) that reach the foetus through the amniotic fluid and the mother's tissues, while high frequencies above 200 Hz are largely filtered and reach a maximum of 40 dB.
7 Day and night rhythm of the mother
8 Rhythmic learning: mother's walking, heartbeat at different speeds, repetition of sounds, moods, movements
9 Being in a fluid medium, being able to feel "fluid" yourself, being able to be in the flow
10 Being able to hover
11 It is predominantly dark, otherwise reddish light, entoptic phenomena are perceptible and the blood vessels on the outside.
12 Blood vessel pattern, root system of the placenta, the "primordial tree" are visible.
13 37 degrees, heat
14 Constant supply via the umbilical cord (nutrients, oxygen, etc.), the abdomen is felt as the central supply point for food and relationship ("gut feeling").
15 Liveliness and moods, feelings of the mother, like inner clouds
16 Taste perception, depending on what the mother has eaten.
17 Experiences of contact with oneself and with and through the uterine wall
18 Attention and loving space or burdened, related or unrelated, in contact or lonely, colourful or grey
19 The mother's hormone messages as grey, mixed or colourful rain, atmosphere, shiver, lightning or touch, as a cloud; the greater the mother's joy, the more colourful the hormone messages, e.g. oxytocin, the more stress or anxiety the mother has (from adrenaline to cortisol), the more split or darker the cloud. Mothers who have orgasmic experiences during

pregnancy communicate to their children that such wonderful feelings exist; prudish mothers are more likely to communicate something sober and uniform about sexuality.

20 Being cocooned in a cave, protected or trapped
21 At the beginning, there is a very large space, but it becomes narrower and narrower; however, this is also an emotional level of the mother's serenity or a narrowness of her fears or constraints.
22 Being able to learn the experience for life, when it gets too tight, you have to get out, something has to be changed (Evertz 2008).

In the mythologies of cultural history, there have always been archetypes of great warmth and love as well as hardship and misery. The myths of mankind's paradise depicted a land flowing with milk and honey. In the myths of hell: distress, fear, panic, shock, proximity to death, powerlessness and agony, when the mother is unwell (illness, trauma, distress, hunger, experience of violence, fear, loneliness, depression, etc.).

In religions, we project these basic patterns onto higher beings and great powers that supposedly have our lives in their hands (Figures 6.4–6.6) (Evertz 2021).

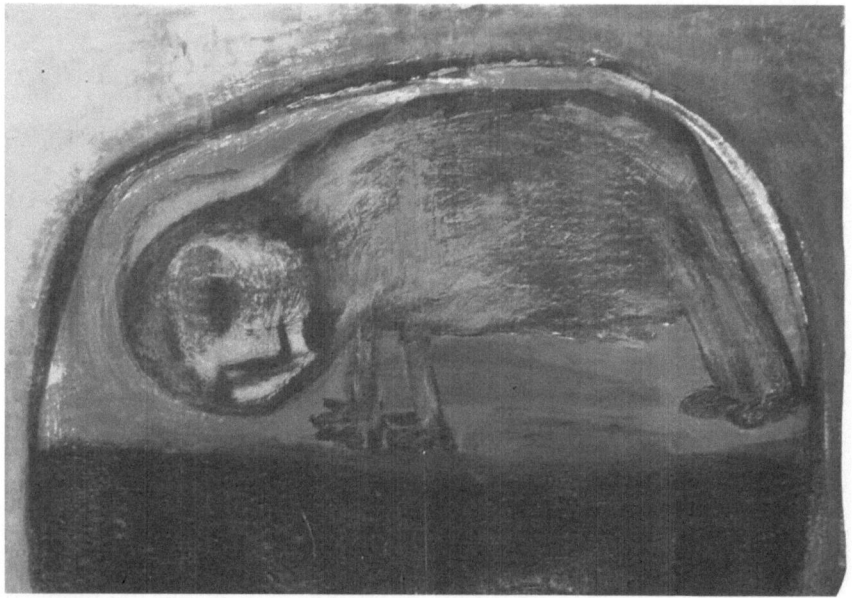

FIGURE 6.4 A picture of a depressed patient who is no longer welcome as the sixth child.

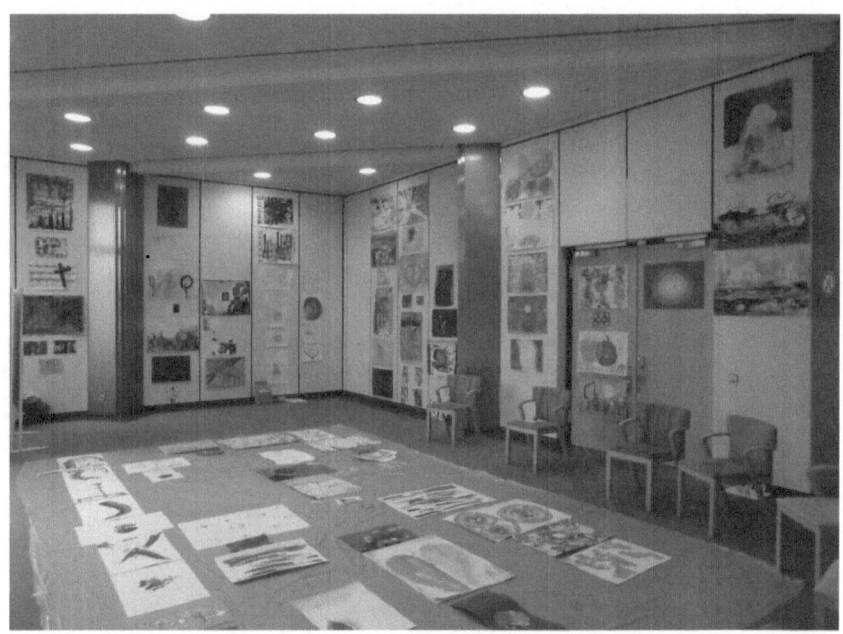

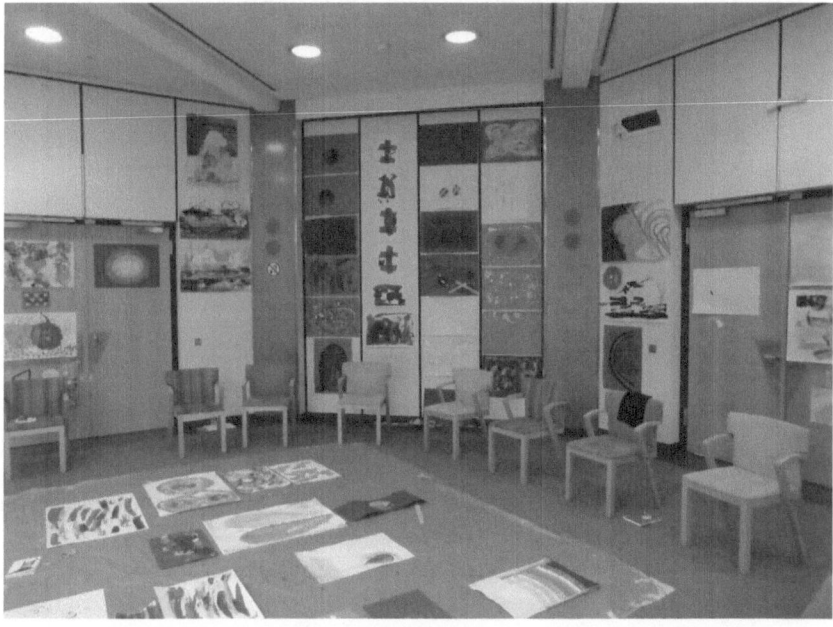

FIGURE 6.5 AND 6.6 Millions of aesthetic formations are painted in deeply regressive art-psychotherapeutic settings. There are always parts of intrauterine primal experiences in paintings.

What do people experience during pregnancy?

It becomes clear that the prenatal patterns of perception are the basis for all postnatal perceptions.

What do we project from our adult perception and our adult consciousness onto this phase of being human? What can we remember? What can we fantasise about it? But even fiction can only ever be the last place of memory.

The Australian music psychologist Parncutt also researches prenatal patterns of perception, which he calls prenatal schemata (Parncutt 2009).

Think of the maternal heartbeat. The cognitive ability to learn patterns is present in the third trimester. The foetus hears the maternal heartbeat for about 20 weeks before it is born at 40 weeks. If it sleeps for 90% of this time and does not process the incoming sounds, and if the heartbeat is inaudible for about half of this time due to other sounds, the foetus will continue to hear the heartbeat for about a week in total. During this time, it has enough time to "learn" how the heartbeat speeds up and slows down, both in cycles linked to the mother's breathing and in the longer term, depending on the mother's physical and emotional state. The foetus also "learns" by association that the variability of the heart rate (speeding up when breathing in and slowing down when breathing out) is higher when the mother is relaxed and lower when she is tense.

Another example is footsteps. If the mother walks for an hour a day (a conservative estimate for a hunter-gatherer) and if the foetus can hear for 20 weeks but sleeps 90% of the time, it will perceive footsteps and associated body movements for a total of 14 hours, allowing it to intuitively learn about the normal speed ranges of footsteps, how isochronous (equally spaced in time) they are compared to the more temporally variable heartbeat sounds, their relationship to foetal body movements, the relationships between their volume and tempo, and the corresponding maternal valence and arousal (reflected in the hormones in the blood if they can be transported through the placenta, and depending on the time delay).

As the mother often speaks or vocalises, the foetus has many opportunities to become familiar with typical fundamental frequency contours and their relationship to the mother's physical and emotional state and breathing. There is a clear relationship between these patterns on the one hand and musical melody and phrasing on the other.

The everyday life of an adult includes emotional highs and lows that correlate with internally audible sounds and movements. Changing hormone concentrations in maternal blood allow the foetus to learn how sound and movement patterns affect the mother's physical and emotional state. Each hormone has different physiological and emotional correlates, and many are lipids that cross the lipid membranes of the placenta and the blood-brain barrier. The time it takes for a change in concentration to cross the placenta (latency) varies.

(Parncutt 2023)

The prenatal situation as a safely enveloped spatial experience, with muffled noises and rhythmic, repetitive, relaxed or excited background basses (the mother's heartbeat) is the archetype of all temples and churches of mankind. They are architectural representations of intrauterine experiences and spaces of longing for – and memory of – warmth, comfort and the highest possible connection and intensity. Just like our enthusiasm to watch the sunsets by the sea, where an "implantation" is performed again and again and thus all our decisions in favour of life (Evertz 2021).

Dance, music and painting as the basic forms of art

The music psychologist Oberhoff described the child's experience in terms of musical tempi: if the mother is relaxing on the couch and taking an afternoon nap, it is a Largo, if the mother is out shopping and strolling, it is an Andante, and if she has to catch the tram quickly and is walking fast, it is a Presto! (Oberhoff 2002)

Music is already one stage more (pre-)symbolic than dance, which is still entirely physical and belongs to the first trimester. In the second trimester, the experience of identity detaches itself from a stronger experience of the outside world and environment. But it also remains close to the direct experience of the body. In the second trimester, the not yet differentiated multipotent neurones migrate to their final locations. The structure of the neuronal network is "fluid", so that aesthetically we can speak of representations as "flowing forms", which can later be found in music in all possible (hormone release) shades, usually underpinned by a "heartbeat" rhythm (Evertz 2015).

- The foetus's sense of hearing is stimulated early on, as there is loud noise in utero from blood flow, heartbeats, bowel sounds, the mother's voice and external noises.
- At 21 weeks, the child reacts to acoustic signals and from 24 weeks onwards can remember the mother's voice, speech melody and spoken words as well as repeatedly heard music. From 32 weeks at the latest, the child prefers certain speech melodies and word sequences from the mother and can be calmed or excited by these. This could be the beginning of learning the mother tongue.
- Important musical elements resemble intrauterine sounds; the rhythm of the music resembles the mother's heartbeat, and string and wind instruments resemble the sounds of blood flow. It is therefore not surprising that music has proved effective in stimulating the foetus and premature babies.

Some authors recommend Beethoven or Mozart but reject rock music (van de Carr 1998). In a study, Linderkamp was able to show that rock music, like quiet music, leads to improved oxygen supply to the brains of premature babies (Linderkamp et al. 2021).

In the third trimester, the representations of flow forms solidify into "persistent and permanent patterns", i.e. the first "stable" feelings/images. This can also be verified by the stabilisation of the bio-chemical-electrical neuronal network in the third trimester of pregnancy. This is where painting (drawing, ultimately all modes of depiction) has its origins.

So there is comprehensive and multisensory perception right from the start! This is how all humans experienced their prenatal period: the arts are ultimately a prenatal developmental psychology in images. We are thus well prepared for a social and relational world because even the intrauterine period was a learning process of social learning and aesthetic perception. We need to take the discussion about the constitution of the self much further into the prenatal space than before and can speak of the competent embryo and foetus.

Summary

Prenatal perception is a comprehensive cosmos of stimulation, touch, development, stimulus demand and contact search and development. The womb is the first space of perception of the world and everything experienced there characterises the later perception of the world. From the very first cell, there is an exchange with the environment and thus a holistic perception that later differentiates into the individual sensory areas during pregnancy but never leaves the synaesthetic ground.

Literature

André V (2018) "The human newborn's environment: Unexplored pathways and perspectives". In: *Psychonomic Bulletin and Review* 25: 350–369.

De Vries JI, Visser GH, Prechtl HF (1982) "The emergence of fetal behaviour. I. Qualitative aspects". In: *Early Human Development* 1982 December; 7(4): 301–322. Doi: 10.1016/0378–3782(82)90033-0.

DiPietro JA (2008) "Prenatal development". In: Haith MM, Benson JB (Editors) *Encyclopedia of infant and early childhood development.* Elsevier, Amsterdam, 604–614.

Evertz K (2008) "Das Bild vor dem Bild - Kunstanalyse, Pränatale Ästhetik und transdisziplinärer Bildbegriff". In: Evertz K, Janus L (eds.) *Kunst als kulturelles Bewusstsein vorgeburtlicher und geburtlicher Erfahrungen.* Mattes, Heidelberg, 85–108.

Evertz K (2015) "Authentizität der Gefühle im künstlerischen Schaffen - Kunstanalyse - Funktionen kreativer Produktion oder das Erkenntnisparadigma der Kunst". In: Kurth W, Janus L (eds.) *Verantwortung für unsere Gefühle - Die emotionale*

Dimension der Aufklärung, Jahrbuch für psychohistorische Forschung, vol. 16. Mattes, Heidelberg, 73–94.

Evertz K (2021) "The prenatal dimension: Images in art and therapy". In: Evertz K et al. (eds.) *Handbook for prenatal psychology - Integrating research and practice*. Springer Nature, Cham, New York, 713–751.

Evertz K (2022) "Die Welt neu spüren – Die transgenerational-systemisch und pränatal fundierte methodenintegrative Psychotherapie – Integrative Kunst- und Körpertherapie". In: Klippel-Heidekrüger M, Janus L (eds.) *Vielfältige Zugänge zum vorsprachlichen und geburtlichen Erleben*, Mattes Verlag, Heidelberg 2022, S. 271–292.

Linderkamp FE, Linderkamp LW, Linderkamp O (2021) "Are music taste and language development influenced by prenatal acoustic experience?" In: Evertz K et al. (eds.) *Handbook for prenatal psychology - Integrating Research and Practice*. Springer Nature, Cham, New York, 701–706.

Oberhoff B (2002) *Psychoanalysis and music*. Psychosozial-Verlag, Giessen.

Parncutt R (2009) "Prenatal development and the phylogeny and ontogeny of musical behavior". In: Hallam S, Cross I, Thaut M (eds.) *Oxford handbook of music psychology*. Oxford University Press, Oxford, 219–228.

Parncutt R (2023) "Pre-linguistic psychology and the origin of man - How the foetus and the fragile infant enabled the emergence of human language, music, art, religion and consciousness". Lecture 28.10.23, ISPPM annual conference "My first universe", Heidelberg.

Van de Carr F.R. (1998) "The Factors in Prenatal and Perinatal Sensory Input", In: nt. J. Prenatal and Perinatal Psychology and Medicine Vol. 10 (1998) No. 4, 477–482

Verny T (2021) *The embodied mind, understanding the mysteries of cellular memory, consciousness and our bodies*. Pegasus Books, New York, London.

7

EMOTIONAL DEVELOPMENT IN THE WOMB

Bonding and relationships

Emotional development can only mean a reciprocal development of attachment and relationship. Pregnancy also means the development of a relationship between three people that was not there before.

However, the relationship between the child and its mother is so physically and emotionally strong that all factors must be taken into consideration. The child learns a great deal about human life and human relationships from its mother. From the very beginning, the child is exposed to all the mother's external and internal movements in the mother's body. It experiences everything. Depending on the mother's emotional mood, it learns its first impressions of love, affection, joy, tenderness, lust, pleasure but also of fear, pain, greed, anger and depression. It offers a cross-section of human passions in an average balance. Its entire organism, its hormone and stress system, develops under these individual conditions. In the bonding analysis, the mother can deepen her contact with the child and shape it more consciously, expressing deep joy and deep fears. The child suffers more from the unspoken and repressed than from the mother's partial avoidance.

If the child receives a lot of positive feedback, it can also develop a healthier self-image and a secure identity. The less feedback they receive, the more difficult it is for them to become a free and independent person.

The fact that we can speak of emotional development in the womb today has a long historical precedent. There have always been cultures that have valued the connection between the generations much more highly than others and that have described contact with the intrauterine child in rituals, music and literature. There have always been cultures that have attributed special possibilities and abilities to being a child because it was closest to

DOI: 10.4324/9781003480242-7

the origin of life, while in other cultures children were only helpless beings and inadequate adults who were simply inferior, who were not fully fledged human beings who could also be killed. The prenatal child has also been recognised or ignored in human history.

Today we know a great deal about the intrauterine child, which has also been aided by the access of increasingly improved ultrasound to pictorial participation in intrauterine life. The photographic images of the child in the womb taken by Nilsson in the 1970s and others have done much to support and stimulate the inner images of adults about their own early life, in addition to research in prenatal medicine and psychology. The perceived images of the beginning of one's own life, widely spread in art and religion, myth and trivial culture, now found a correlate in direct visualisation. The simultaneous safe-guarding of pregnancy and birth processes in gynaecology and neonatology in industrialised countries also took away the fear of being able to look into a phase of life that was often threatened in earlier centuries and often enough ended with the death of the child or even the mother.

But even with the new images of ultrasound and invasive photography, it is important to differentiate the possibilities of fantasies about intrauterine existence from possible real levels of memory. Memory and remembrance discourses in psychology and psychotherapy are very interesting and excit-ing. They range from the impossibility of being able to remember anything at all from early life up to the age of three, which is claimed by representatives of exclusively neocortical research, to religious and esoteric models of foetal omniscience and cosmic consciousness.

Prenatal psychology is taking part in this discourse but with new argu-ments and in a new balance:

1 The baby in its mother's womb is not a superhuman, a saint or a being capable of special wisdom. It doesn't "know" anything at first.
2 But it "knows" something on a level of the physical self that we are only slowly approaching philosophically, scientifically and psychologically.
3 It "knows" something about how life actually works cellularly and molecu-larly and it "knows" something about the fact that life does not exist in vain (Weatherbee 2024).

How should we categorise the indisputable fact that all living beings are part of an evolutionary chain and carry condensed information from all previous generations?

What should we call the "knowledge" that the totipotent cell of our ontogenetic beginnings sets in motion all subsequent developments in its possibilities and abilities? How does the cell "know" how the heart, the eye, the ear, the brain, the limbs and the other organs and systems should develop?

What should we call the biological exchange between mother and child, e.g. during the implantation process, if the mother's immune system does not fight the foreign cell but allows it? What should we call this process of immune tolerance, especially when we have the information that two-thirds of pregnancies already end here? (Weatherbee 2024).

Prenatal medical research has investigated the correlations that pregnancies are more at risk if the couple's emotional relationship dynamics are rather dysfunctional. Prenatal psychology, for its part, has similar research findings. Over 100 years ago, Ferenczi wrote an article on "The unwelcome child and its death instinct". According to his therapeutic observations, adults who came from unhappy relationships were on average also more susceptible to illness and unfit for life and suffered more from somatic and mental disorders and had a lower life expectancy.

In a nutshell, the idea is that a bio-psycho-social view of human beings can understand every form of influence and exchange of information in and between living systems as a form of "knowledge" and "consciousness". In contrast to everyday consciousness, Freud formulated the concept of the unconscious to describe something that takes place below and above all conscious life but which arises from it. In other words, our everyday consciousness is only possible, thanks to an infinite amount of information that should not be conscious, so that we can focus our attention on new things and new developments in everyday life. Evolution is interested in development, not stagnation.

During pregnancy, a woman's body changes in various ways. Some of these changes include

1 Hormonal changes: The body produces an increased amount of hormones such as oestrogen and progesterone to support the pregnancy.
2 Increase in blood volume: A woman's blood volume increases during pregnancy in order to supply the growing baby with sufficient nutrients and oxygen.
3 Changes in the breasts: The breasts may become larger and more sensitive as they prepare to produce breast milk.
4 Weight gain: The woman gains weight during pregnancy as the baby develops and grows.
5 Changes in the digestive system: Many women experience digestive problems such as heartburn or constipation during pregnancy due to the pressure of the growing baby on the organs.
6 Dilation of the uterus: The uterus expands to make room for the growing baby.
7 Changes in the skin: Many women experience changes in their skin during pregnancy, such as changes in pigmentation or the appearance of stretch marks.

These are just a few examples of the many changes that can occur in a woman's body during pregnancy. Each pregnancy is unique and can have different effects on the body. These changes indicate the magnitude of the transformation process that the woman undergoes during pregnancy and that she undergoes with the child growing inside her bio-psycho-socially, i.e. also emotionally. For example, the quickening, when a pregnant person begins to feel the movements of the baby in her womb. It feels like fluttering, bubbles or tiny pulses. Quickening occurs around the 16th–20th week of pregnancy but can also occur earlier or later.

The emotional development of the child in the womb during pregnancy can be divided into different phases. It is important to note that the exact sequence and duration of these phases can vary from individual to individual, but that in any case it is about a real, rich emotional-sensory world of the intrauterine child.

1 Earliest phase: All cell development processes are moulding processes from which later developments emerge. Cell memory is evident.
2 Early phase: The emotional development of the foetus begins in the first few weeks of pregnancy. Although the nervous system is not yet fully developed, the first signs of emotional response can be observed. The foetus can react to certain stimuli, such as touch or loud noises.
3 Sensitisation phase: In the second trimester of pregnancy, the foetus' sensitivity to external stimuli increases. The foetus can react to stimuli from the environment, such as the mother's voice or gentle touches on the abdomen. These reactions can become visible through movements or changes in the foetus's heartbeat.
4 Interaction phase: In the third trimester of pregnancy, the foetus' ability to interact with its environment continues to develop. The foetus can respond to different types of stimulation and may show preferences for certain stimuli or activities. For example, the child may become calmer when it hears the mother's voice or move when it is gently stroked.
5 Preparation phase: Towards the end of pregnancy, the child prepares for birth and life outside the womb. The foetus can react more strongly to the mother's movements and positions, as this has an effect on its own body. During this phase, the foetus reacts particularly noticeably to the mother's emotional states, such as stress or relaxation.

It is important to note that the emotional development of the child in the womb during pregnancy is still the subject of intensive research and many aspects remain to be explored. The exact nature and meaning of the foetus' emotional experiences are not yet fully understood, but we do know that they have an impact on the child's later emotional development.

Attachment and relationship – father, mother, child – primal bond and primal trust

Pregnancy is an event involving three people: mother, father and child. Of course, the mother and child are in a bio-psycho-social bond of exclusivity, closeness and physical symbiosis that will hardly be found later in relationships between people. However, many of our projections of longing for love between man and woman are characterised by the desire to achieve the highest intensity of closeness again. Our entire art and trivial culture is centred on the theme of love, lust, pain and death. Just listen to the hit lists of pop culture.

This great exclusive intimate relationship between mother and child is therefore the archetype of all great human concepts of love. The father seems to be further away. In reality, however, pregnancy is about triangulation, a relationship between three people. The more the father is involved in the developing relationship with the child through the mother's inner images, the more fulfilling the feeling of love between mother and child. Indeed, the mother can only build a clear object relationship with the child if she has strong and positive images of the man with whom she fathered the child (Raffai 2014).

During the course of the pregnancy, the child can "feel" this third party of the father not only through the hereditary part, as half of the DNA comes from the father but also through the emotional quality of communication between the father and mother during the pregnancy. In a certain sense, the child senses how the mother reacts to the father right from the start, more clearly and sensually from the second trimester onwards. It senses the mother's changing behaviour and excitement when the father is nearby, it hears the father's voice alongside the mother's voice and senses the changes in the atmosphere when the two are a happy couple and spend time together.

Of course, the child also feels the mother's pain and sadness if the couple is not happy, e.g. if the father leaves the mother and leaves her alone with the task of growing the child inside her and bringing it into the world. The child also senses the quarrels of unhappy couples and, like the mother, closes off when there is a lot of fear, violence and dissatisfaction in the relationship.

One of the first important studies in prenatal psychology was the Scandinavian study by Huttunen and Niskanen (1978), where severe personality disorders in psychiatric patients were attributed to the loss of the father during pregnancy (Figure 7.1). The immeasurable pain of a pregnant woman when her husband is killed in an accident or dies of an illness understandably leads to such severe dysfunction that the intrauterine child's sense of self is so permanently shaken by this traumatic disturbance that severe personality disorders are more likely later on (Raffai 2014, 2021).

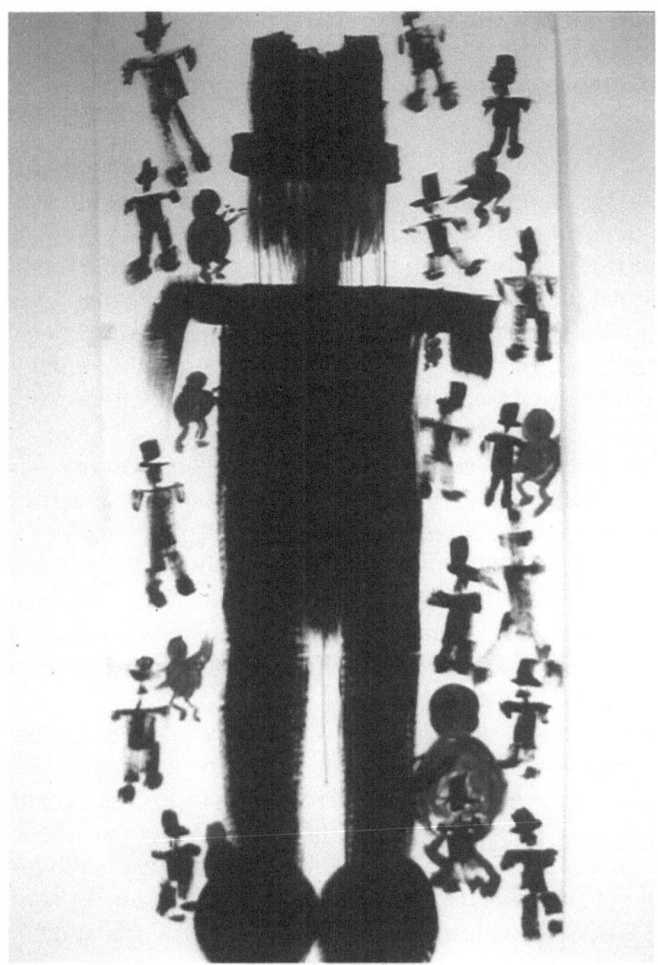

FIGURE 7.1   Large picture of a 30-year-old doctor whose father was diagnosed with leukaemia when she was three months pregnant. The father then died six weeks after her birth. Her pregnancy was therefore burdened by her mother's panic that her husband would soon die. The client was unable to build a deeper relationship with a man until the therapy.

A major misfortune during pregnancy is therefore also a particular risk factor for the child's later life but also a special opportunity. Bill Clinton also lost his father during his prenatal period. Later becoming President of the United States can also be seen as an extraordinary feat of energy, transforming a trauma into a talent. He had to emotionally support his mother during his pregnancy and was thus able to learn how to take responsibility for such a huge system as the most powerful country on earth.

The development of a theory of prenatal bonding

Prenatal bonding – maternal–foetal bonding – paternal–foetal bonding

The theory of prenatal bonding has a complex developmental history. Here, too, there are two strands that have developed in parallel. One strand, which is also the older one, developed from observation in a psychoanalytical or psychotherapeutic setting. Here the researcher enters into a therapeutic and/ or psychosocial relationship with the couple or the pregnant woman or the adult patient suffering from somatic or psychological disorders originating in early childhood, birth and pregnancy. The therapeutic relationship takes precedence over any research goals and is usually depth-psychological and qualitatively observational (Janus 2000).

The second strand is research involving quantitative observation and interviews with pregnant couples. Here the researcher only acts as a researcher or in low-threshold psychosocial counselling. Brandon (2009) provides a good overview of this second field of research. She lists observational non-therapeutic research and discusses the possibilities of extending Bowlby's attachment theory into the prenatal area. A small selection of studies will suffice here:

Lumley conducted semi-structured interviews with first-time parents.

> The degree of foetal development was greatly underestimated in the first trimester. By mid-pregnancy, ideas about the foetus became more accurate and all women gave very realistic descriptions by 36 weeks. Although most women in early pregnancy had difficulty believing that the foetus really existed, a minority had an attachment to the baby by the 8th to 12th week. Maternal "attachment" to the foetus was detectable in 63% of women at 18 to 22 weeks' gestation and in 92% at 36 weeks' gestation.
>
> *(Lumley 1982, p. 106)*

Cranley developed a scale to assess prenatal attachment, the Maternal–Foetal Attachment Scale (MFAS). The following levels of attachment are examined: the assumption of the mother's role, contact with the foetus, the perception of characteristics of the foetus and the distinction between the maternal self and the foetus (Cranley 1981).

Condon investigated even more specifically and called his scale the "Maternal Antenatal Attachment Scale – MAAS". The focus is on the mother's feelings and thoughts about the baby. Protection, security, separation and loss, the child's needs and their fulfilment are at the forefront.

> The type of relationship that expectant parents develop with their unborn child during pregnancy has both theoretical and clinical significance.

It potentially provides a framework for a better understanding of many aspects of psychosomatic obstetrics, including responses to foetal loss. Existing tools for assessing this relationship do not adequately distinguish between attitudes towards the foetus per se and attitudes towards the state of pregnancy or maternal role. In this paper, a theoretical model of the subjective experience of human attachment is presented. This model is used to develop a questionnaire to assess the construct of prenatal attachment. Item analysis results in a 19 item maternal and 16 item paternal questionnaire with high internal consistency. Each questionnaire takes about five minutes to complete. Finally, the factor structures of the resulting questionnaires are analysed.

(Condon 1993, p. 167)

Ammaniti and Gallese researched maternal perceptions of the child during pregnancy and developed three models from clinical observations:

1 The integrated/balanced representation model
2 The restricted/disinvested representation model
3 The non-integrated/ambivalent representation model

The first model, which is the most common, is an integrated concept of motherhood in which the child is recognised and loved as a new being in its own right. The successful relationship with the child is characterised by strong emotional involvement, openness and flexibility. It corresponds to Raffai's (2014, 2021) observation of a clear, healthy object relationship even before birth, through which the child already feels reflected and accepted and can form its own physical boundaries instead of blurring with the mother or being symbiotically constricted by her projections.

The second model describes pregnancies in which emotional control is dominant and rationalisations towards motherhood and the child prevail. There are few images and fantasies and dreams, little vitality towards a creative human being.

The third model is characterised by contradictory and distorting attitudes on the part of the mother and essentially also by authority-fixated parents who have not yet detached themselves from their own parents.

Risk factors during pregnancy were most likely to occur in the second and third models (Ammaniti & Gallese 2014).

So while Bowlby and his colleagues proved how important attentive and empathetic care for infants and young children is for lifelong mental health, prenatal attachment research goes further and can prove that the foundations for lifelong mental health already lie in pregnancy.

The importance of prenatal bonding

Quantitative–qualitative research on prenatal bonding has pursued its objectives and differentiated the levels:

- During pregnancy, mothers can develop their ability to care and learn to become mothers.
- From a clinical perspective, the concept of prenatal bonding therefore makes it easier to describe the emotional experience of pregnancy.
- Expanding clinical understanding of the psychological cost of foetal loss
- Women who are unsure of their attachment can respond to appropriate interventions.
- Women who are not aware of or do not care about their attachment to the foetus can benefit from education and motivation.
- The mother's conscious awareness of the baby's movements, e.g. counting the number of movements she feels and responding by tapping the abdominal wall the same number of times, significantly strengthens the maternal–foetal bond (Mikhail et al. 1991).
- The intergenerational quality of attachment becomes a topic of investigation (Fonagy et al. 1991).
- Secure mothers have secure babies, insecure mothers have insecure babies: it becomes possible to address families with insecure attachment styles and develop interventions (Priel & Besser 2000).

(cf. Brandon 2009, p. 216f).

Poor attachment has also been linked to the painful issue of foetal and infant abuse. An English study of a sample of 40 women referred by social services found that 'negatively anxious' antenatal attachment (as measured by the Maternal Antenatal Attachment Scale) increased the likelihood of anxiety symptoms, mood disorders and depression, self-reported fetal irritation and even fetal maltreatment (Pollock & Percy 1999). Other researchers have examined the relationship between insecure attachment in mothers and the incidence of child abuse and found positive correlations (Moncher 1996). In contrast, strong MFA has been associated with positive health practices during pregnancy, such as abstinence from tobacco, alcohol and illicit drugs, use of prenatal care, healthy diet and sleep habits, adequate exercise, seatbelt use, and learning about pregnancy, birth and infant care (Lindgren 2001).

(Brandon 2009, p. 216f)

Prenatal attachment theory states that a unique relationship develops between parents and foetus long before the child is born. Since its introduction in the 1970s by a few key individuals, primarily nurses, measures of prenatal attachment have been developed to assess maternal and paternal fetal bonding. Research has shown that prenatal attachment motivates good health behaviours during pregnancy, facilitates adjustment to the parental role and may even serve as a protective factor against perinatal depression. This makes this theoretical approach to pregnancy important in all academic and clinical disciplines of medicine, psychiatry and social work. As research into attachment disorders continues, new importance is being placed on early detection and intervention.

Ideally, additional knowledge about the role of the MFA could promote the development of interventions that begin before birth and prevent poor mother-infant bonding from being an 'inevitable sequence of events'.

(Brandon 2009, p. 218)

The 2021 study 'Pregnancy Intendedness, Maternal-Fetal Bonding, and Postnatal Maternal-Infant Bonding' further complements this research.

(Shreffler et al. 2021)

The therapeutic qualitative exploration of prenatal bonding

Therapeutic qualitative research can only confirm the above findings but goes even further in differentiating the psychodynamics of the parents-to-be and the maternal–foetal and paternal–foetal bond:

- The wanted or unwanted nature of pregnancy
- The couple dynamics of the parents
- Functionality or dysfunctionality of the two family systems
- The traumas of the two family systems and psychosocial stress or trauma during pregnancy
- Psychosocial stress during pregnancy
- Diseases during pregnancy and pregnancy complications

Frank Lake explored Maternal-Fetal Distress Syndrome (M-FDS) as a new and far-reaching paradigm in counselling. "The main thesis is that a prenatal environment exists at conception, followed by a week of happy "union" and unattachment (the blastocyst stage), then implantation occurs, and a mother-baby bond develops during pregnancy. The first trimester of intrauterine life is the source of profound imprints that affect the entire adult life….

According to Lake, the bidirectional flow of the "navel effect" between the mother and her unborn child can lead to three relationship patterns based on the mother's positive, negative or strongly negative emotions. The mother's emotions inspire four variations of foetal response, ranging from the 'ideal' state of warm and connected happiness to 'coping', 'opposition' (aggressively active to passively non-cooperative) and 'transmarginal stress' (a catastrophic state in which 'the self turns against itself'). Here lie the roots of maternal-fetal stress syndrome, which creates a psycho-physiological predisposition for personality disorders or psychosomatic symptoms. These forces can also complicate pregnancy and labour. For Lake, there is also an ontology of the normal mother-child relationship based on two input phases (being/well-being) and two output phases (status/achievement) at each stage of development. These in turn affect the subsequent exchange relationships.

(https://birthpsychology.com/book-review/prenatal-person-frank-lakeaposs-maternal-fetal-distress-syndrome)

These observations coincide with Catherine Monk's biopsychological research:

Catherine Monk, a psychologist at Columbia University, New York, is conducting a long-term study to investigate how pregnant women and their children react to stress. In the so-called Stroop test, the test subjects have to solve tasks on the computer under time pressure. The results show that blood pressure, respiratory rate and heart rate rose sharply in all pregnant women. However, the heart rate of the intrauterine foetus only increased in the test subjects who suffered from previously untreated anxiety disorders or depression. These foetuses are therefore noticeably more sensitive to stress than others. This pattern continues after birth: the babies are more nervous and less easily calmed than their peers (Monk et al. 2016; Koch 2012).

> Monk suspects a mechanism for the phenomenon at the molecular level. It is possible that maternal melancholy leads to changes in the gene expression of certain proteins in the placenta. Normally, the placenta serves as a kind of protective barrier that keeps harmful substances away from the child. Enzymes are active in its cells that can at least partially neutralise stress hormones. If these are disabled, Monk believes, the mother's cortisol, for example, reaches the child in much higher concentrations.
>
> *(Koch 2012, p. 128)*

What sounds so relatively trivialised in the "technical" language of medicine and biology can, however, be very panicky and frightening for an intrauterine child in reality, depending on the extent of the maternal stress (Figures 7.2 and 7.3). The following picture shows something of the reality of the experience when an adult patient tries to visualise the intrauterine stress, which in a certain sense has never stopped for her (Evertz 2020, 2021a).

Wonderful images of the intrauterine period thus stand alongside catastrophic images. Cultural history shows us a wealth of qualities of prenatal bonding between images of paradise and hell, which we can increasingly

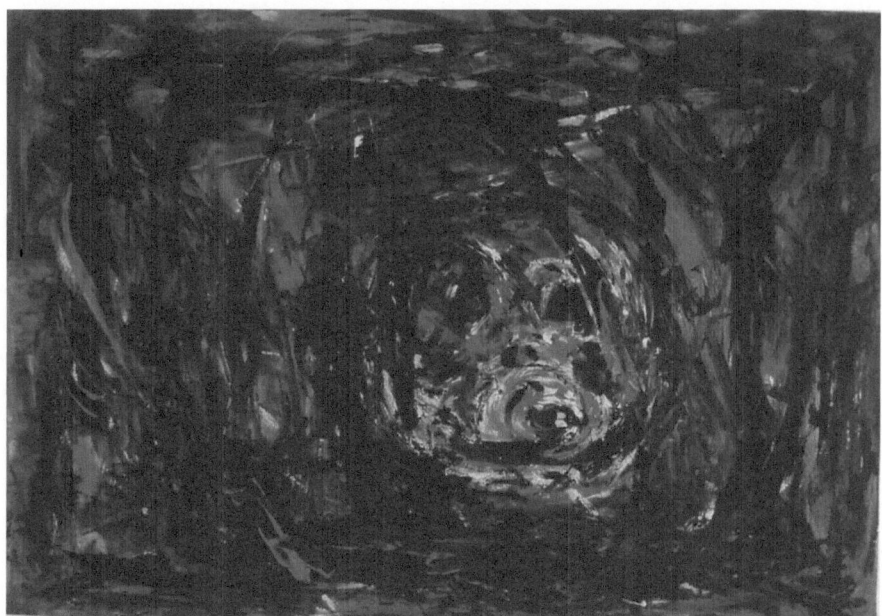

FIGURE 7.2   Painting of a patient with a complex mental illness with the theme of intrauterine hopelessness in the womb of the depressed mother.

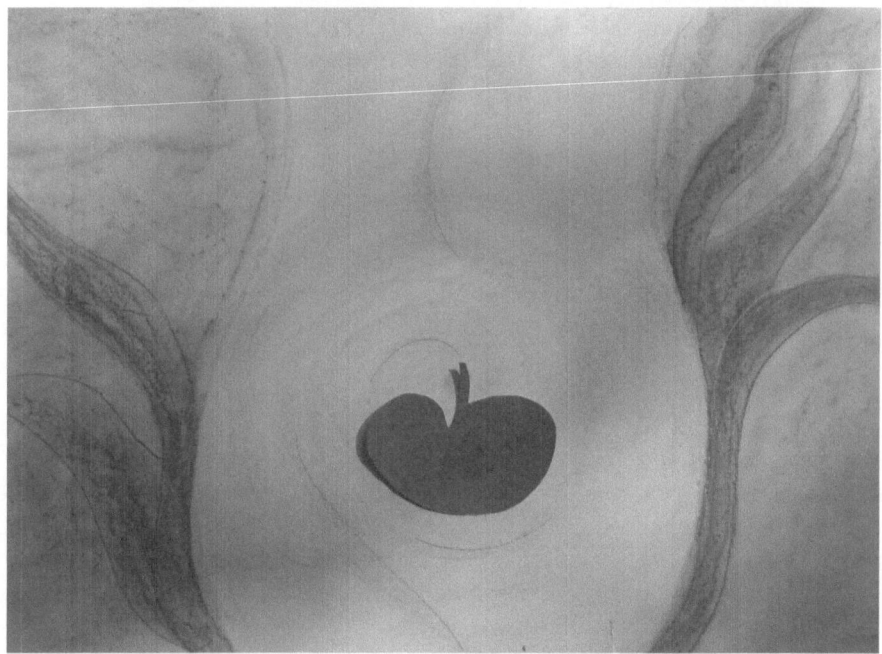

FIGURE 7.3   Painting by a training participant: being seen and loved.

learn to read as collective memory atmospheres of the pregnancy experiences of thousands of generations (Janus & Evertz 2008; Evertz 2021b).

The spectrum of prenatal bonding therefore lies between primal experiences of wonderful love and primal experiences of the greatest fear. In the first case, the baby is a much-loved new creature that needs to be protected and given every opportunity to enjoy life, be raised and educated; in the second case, it can be a kind of parasite or alien that eats the mother from the inside and destroys her life. The worldwide success of Ridley Scott's "Alien" films shows the ubiquitous fantasy of the experience of pregnancy as a murderous and toxic event in the life of a previously traumatised woman who is unable to develop her female potential.

The qualitatively biographical and transgenerationally more extensive research strand of prenatal psychology thus develops the theory of prenatal attachment from the experiences in the depth-psychological setting, which can take into account the entire spectrum of human experience (see also Chapters 2, 4–6, 8 and 9 in this book).

A very valuable contribution to prenatal attachment research is the method of attachment analysis, which was developed by the Hungarian psychoanalysts Raffai and Hidas (Hidas & Raffai 2006). The prophylactic work of attachment analysis was developed from the psychoanalytical observation that pregnant mothers can have very different representations of their child and very different feelings about their pregnancy, which can result in very complex imprints on the child's life. It is intended to help strengthen the mother's feelings and emotions towards her child during pregnancy and make her more aware of them in order to improve and support the bond between mother and child.

> Bonding analysis or prenatal bonding (BA) helps the pregnant woman to connect with her still unborn baby and opens up opportunities for two-way communication. The mother can enter into an inner dialogue with her baby that was previously not considered possible by obstetricians, medical professionals and psychologists. The developing communication patterns are the basis for a growing emotional bond and enable mother and baby to cope with the birth as a team.
>
> *(Goertz-Schroth et al. 2023, p. 1)*

This very empathetic attachment analysis work, which is not actually therapeutic in nature but has a therapeutic background, takes into account the mother's need to be recognised in her strength as well as in her fears. The mother's feelings and emotions, whether and how she communicates with her child, are sensitively accompanied and the spectrum of perception of broad interaction possibilities is expanded.

In a retrospective study, the birth outcomes of 295 women who were accompanied during their pregnancy with Bonding Analysis/Prenatal

Bonding (BA) were analysed. The results show that the need for obstetric interventions and caesarean sections decreased and breastfeeding rates increased. Premature births, insatiable crying and postpartum depression were extremely rare. As the mother and her newborn were able to bond before birth, the postnatal period became an encouraging phase in the development of an existing relationship.

(Goertz-Schroth et al. 2023, p. 1)

Attachment analysis as a particularly effective psychosocial intervention

Prenatal attachment analysis (prenatal bonding (BA)) is a method that aims to examine and promote the relationship between parents and their unborn child. Here is a list of aspects that can be considered in a prenatal attachment analysis:

1 Pregnancy history: The analysis may include information about the course of the pregnancy, medical examinations and possible risk factors.
2 Emotional attachment: The emotional bond between the parents and the unborn child is analysed. This can be determined through interviews, questionnaires or conversations.
3 Communication: The way in which the parents communicate with each other and with the unborn child is analysed. This includes both verbal and non-verbal communication.
4 Physical closeness: The analysis can examine how much physical closeness and touch there is between the parents and the unborn child.
5 Fears and worries: It is determined whether there are fears or worries that could influence the bond. These could be, for example, fears about the birth or insecurities about the parental role.
6 Preparation for the birth: The analysis can also examine how the parents are preparing for the upcoming birth and what their expectations are.
7 Support systems: We look at the support systems available to parents, such as family, friends or professional help.
8 Attachment history: The analysis can also take into account the parents' individual attachment history and examine how this influences their relationship with the unborn child.
9 Stress factors: It is determined whether there are stress factors that could impair the bond, such as financial problems or family conflicts.
10 Resources and strengths: We look at what resources and strengths the parents have to build and maintain a positive bond with their unborn child.

It is important to note that a prenatal attachment analysis should be carried out by qualified professionals who have knowledge in this area. The results of such an analysis can help to strengthen the relationship between parents and their unborn child and recognise potential challenges at an early stage.

The psychoanalyst and attachment analyst Schroth writes:

> Medical progress in recent decades has improved the safety of pregnancy, birth and early childhood. Nevertheless, maternal and infant mortality rates have not fallen to the extent needed to achieve UNICEF's Sustainable Development Goals for 2030 (UNFPA 2019; UNICEF 2023). This indicates that more should be done to optimise maternal and infant care.
>
> Researchers have proven the connection between emotional and physical well-being, and a growing part of medicine is applying this knowledge to pregnancy and birth. Kennell and Klaus demonstrated that the presence of a doula during labour is associated with a significant reduction in caesarean births (Kennell et al. 1991).
>
> Fredrick Leboyer argued in favour of looking at birth from the baby's perspective and designing obstetric care in such a way that the baby is supported in a gentle and natural birth (Conley 2010). Bowlby and Ainsworth investigated the effects of secure or insecure mother–infant attachment on infants and young children and developed an attachment theory (Bretherton 1992). Phillips has described how uninterrupted skin-to-skin contact immediately after vaginal birth and caesarean delivery promotes mother–infant bonding and increases breastfeeding rates, which has been shown to improve maternal and infant outcomes (Centers for Disease Control and Prevention [CDC] 2021; Phillips 2012, 2013). There is growing evidence that maternal mental health during pregnancy has a direct impact on foetal and child development (Jeličić et al. 2022; Molenaar et al. 2019; Simons et al. 2019; Van den Bergh et al. 2020; Wu et al. 2022).
>
> *(Goertz-Schroth et al. 2023, p. 3)*

For more than 100 years, pre- and perinatal psychology has suggested that understanding and supporting the mental health of mother and baby during pregnancy improves birth outcomes (Evertz 2021; Janus 2021). In the 1970s, Thomas Verny, a Canadian psychiatrist, and David Chamberlain, a US psychologist, discovered in their respective therapeutic settings that many children and adults have memories of the time before, during and after birth - often with profound long-term effects on their lives (Chamberlain 1988; Verny & Kelly 1981). Verny and Chamberlain independently discovered that mental disorders associated with these traumas often resolved when traumatic experiences before or during birth or infancy were treated through hypnosis or other psychotherapeutic techniques. The realisation that prenatal and birth memories are stored in the unconscious and in body memory was groundbreaking and led to new methods of early preverbal trauma management.

This knowledge not only provided new information about the prenatal psyche, but also raised awareness of the possibility of an emotional connection between the pregnant mother and the unborn child. It has been known since the 1990s that the mother-child bond is crucial for normal development (Bretherton 1992). However, it was previously assumed that bonding would only begin after birth. The groundbreaking realisation that emotional bonding can begin before birth opened up new, previously unimagined possibilities for supporting pregnancy, birth, early postnatal development of the child and the family.

Pregnancy counsellors encouraged expectant mothers to talk to their babies, sing and imagine how their baby was growing and developing in the womb. It was assumed that this interaction would only go in one direction. Many mothers began to talk to their babies, but few realised that they could receive feedback from their unborn babies while they were still in the womb.

(Goertz-Schroth et al. 2023, p. 4)

The results of the first study on the application of attachment analysis are so significant that they are reproduced here in full:

Premature births

292 pregnant women (99%) gave birth to their babies at term (37 to 42 weeks' gestation) while 3 babies (1%) were born late preterm. Two mothers (0.7%) gave birth in the 36th week of pregnancy and 1 mother (0.3%) gave birth in the 34th week.

Mode of birth

227 women (77%) went into labour spontaneously and 94 women (32%) gave birth without medication or other obstetric interventions. 82% of the women gave birth vaginally. A caesarean section was deemed necessary by the doctors in 53 births (18%).

Place of birth

A total of 261 births (88.5%) took place in a hospital, 30 births (10.2%) at home and 4 births (1.3%) in a birthing centre.

Breastfeeding

292 mothers (99%) successfully started breastfeeding and only 3 women (1%) were unable to breastfeed after giving birth. A further 15 women

(5%) were only able to breastfeed partially, i.e. they breastfed with complementary foods or for less than six months. At the age of six months, 277 infants (94%) were still being breastfed.

Screaming and crying

Only one baby (0.3%) out of 295 was a so-called "cry baby" according to the applicable criteria. In 2 other cases (0.7%), the baby cried for 30–60 minutes per day in the first few weeks.

Postpartum depression

While 292 women (99%) were completely free of symptoms of postpartum depression, three mothers (1%) experienced some symptoms.

Baby blues

18 mothers (6%) suffered from symptoms of the baby blues for a maximum of two weeks, while 277 mothers (94%) were completely symptom-free.

(Goertz-Schroth et al. 2023, p. 5)

Discussion

This retrospective study shows that the birth outcomes of mothers and infants are significantly more favourable after support with attachment analysis/prenatal bonding (BA) than with unaccompanied pregnant women (Goertz-Schroth et al. 2023).

Pregnancy ambivalences

The wanted child and the unwanted child, abortion fantasies, abortion attempts, artificial insemination

Whether external reasons or internal motives are decisive in a pregnancy conflict situation, unconscious, sometimes transgenerational dynamics can usually be recognised more clearly in psychotherapy and included in the considerations. Delivery, miscarriage, premature birth, stillbirth and abortion are often not so far apart. In order to finally make the unspeakable discussions about guilt in the context of pregnancy conflicts superfluous, it is necessary to include the psychodynamic level and to place the question of the difficulties and beauties of passing on life on a broader and more humane level.

In contrast to normal conflict counselling, in psychotherapy with a pregnant client, we have the opportunity to address much deeper levels of the psychodynamics of the conflict. Conversely, only a few women and couples in a pregnancy conflict have so far sought out a psychotherapeutic practice, let alone men alone.

Unconscious abortive tendencies often stem from unresolved pre- and perinatal and early childhood traumas of the expectant parents or transgenerational conflicts in the family. Abortion is often an emergency solution to unbearable unconscious pain, horror and anguish. Due to the couple's deep fear of having to kill the child later, the embryo has to be aborted. The real child in the uterus is confused with the traumatised "inner child" of the father or mother. These processes are essentially unconscious, but strongly motivate action, and are very complex and therefore hardly ever appear in public discussion (Evertz 2021a).

Globally, sex-selective abortion, the practice of terminating a pregnancy based on the expected sex of the child, is a major population and health policy problem. Parents want a child but only if it is male. The selective abortion of female foetuses is particularly common where male children are valued more highly than female children, especially in parts of East and South Asia. In other words, especially in cultures that are still patriarchal and where women's rights are not yet recognised (Hesketh et al. 2011).

An as-yet unpublished study by a counselling centre for pregnant women in Berlin shows the cross-section of reasons for terminating a pregnancy, as can be heard in daily consultations worldwide (Figure 7.4).

The issue of abortion is a complex and controversial one, involving various ethical, legal and health aspects. Here are some of the key issues surrounding abortion:

1 Right to bodily autonomy: A central issue in the abortion debate is a woman's right to bodily autonomy and self-determination over her own body. Advocates argue that women should have the right to decide about pregnancy and have access to safe and legal abortions.
2 Foetal rights: One counter-argument to abortion is based on the protection of the rights of the unborn child. Opponents argue that a foetus is an independent life and therefore has the right to life, which should not be violated. Furthermore, abortionists have claimed the right to life for themselves and are denying it to others.
3 Health effects: The health effects of abortion are also important. Advocates argue that access to safe and legal abortions protects women's health by preventing unwanted pregnancies and reducing complications from unsafe practices.
4 Religious and moral convictions: The issue of abortion is also often influenced by religious or moral beliefs. Some religions view abortion as morally wrong or sinful, while others emphasise the protection of bodily autonomy.

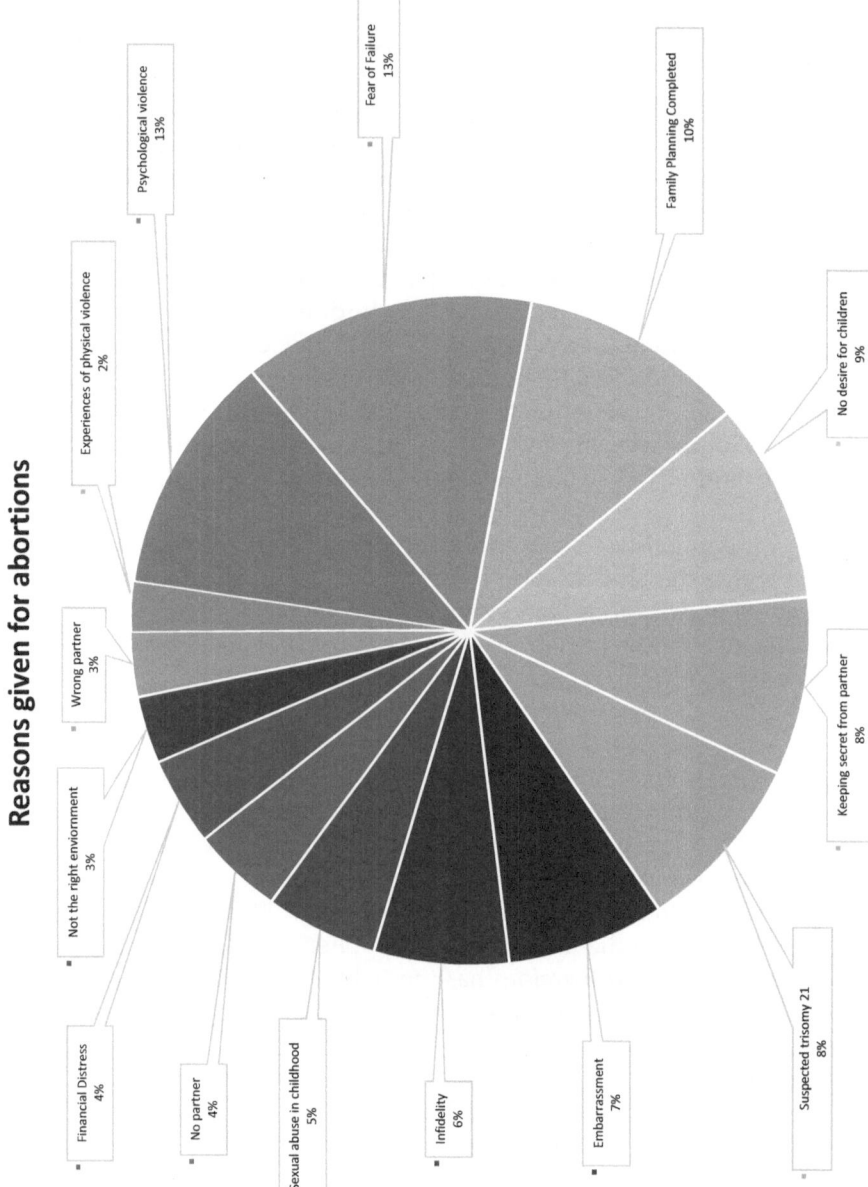

FIGURE 7.4 Reasons for abortions (Müller 2020, p. 14).

5 Legislation and access: The legal regulation of abortion varies from country to country and can affect access to safe and legal procedures. Legislative issues include the regulation of time limits, the availability of abortion for medical indications and the role of counselling services.
6 Sexual education and contraception: Another important aspect of the abortion debate is the promotion of sexual education and contraception to prevent unwanted pregnancies. Advocates argue that better access to contraception and sex education can help to reduce the number of abortions.
7 Post-abortion care: Support and care for women after an abortion is also important. This includes psychological support, medical aftercare and access to family planning and contraceptive services.

It is important to note that this list only covers some of the many issues surrounding abortion. Views on this topic are diverse and can vary widely. It is advisable to read up on local laws, policies and ethical considerations to form an informed opinion (Linder 2021).

A case study of a 45-year-old cancer patient who was able to access her primal trauma of a survived abortion attempt through art-psychotherapeutic processes and who experienced sustainable healing processes (Figures 7.5– 7.8).

Artificial insemination

Artificial insemination, also known as assisted reproductive technology (ART), involves various procedures to assist reproduction in couples with fertility problems. Here are some important facts about artificial insemination:

1 Success rate: The success rate of artificial insemination varies depending on the method used and the individual circumstances of the couple. In vitro fertilisation (IVF) is one of the most common ART methods and has a success rate of around 30–40% per cycle for women under the age of 35.
2 Causes of infertility: Artificial insemination can help with various causes of infertility, such as problems with the fallopian tubes, low sperm count or quality, endometriosis or hormonal disorders. The psychological background usually also reveals the deeper conflicts behind infertility.
3 Multiple pregnancies: One of the challenges of artificial insemination is to minimise the risk of multiple pregnancies. The use of single embryo transfer (one embryo transfer per cycle) has helped to reduce the rate of multiple pregnancies.
4 Genetic tests: Genetic tests can be carried out before the transfer to identify certain genetic diseases or chromosomal abnormalities and minimise the risk for the child.

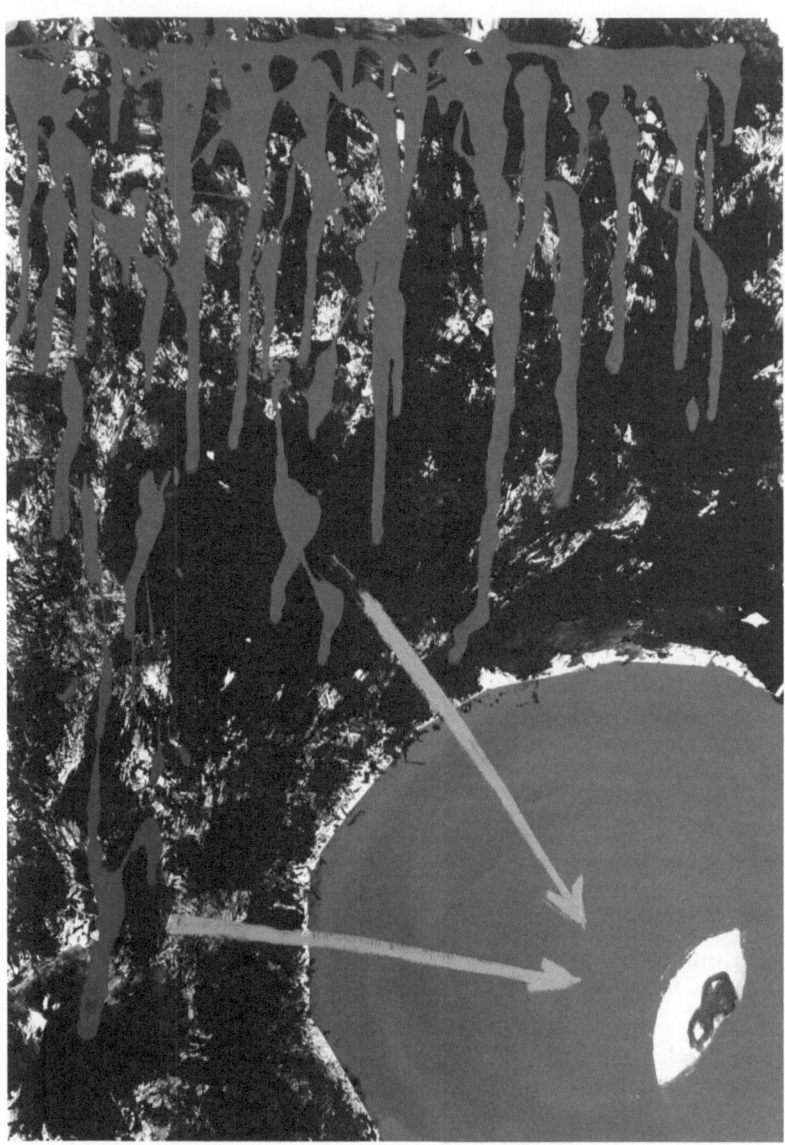

FIGURE 7.5 Picture 1 In a group workshop, a 45-year-old cancer patient paints a picture of her mother's attempted abortion with needles during her embryonic period (image 1). In a second picture, she paints the split resulting from this trauma, which determined her life for over 40 years as a sequence of many relationship disasters (picture 2). In a third picture, she arrives at the aesthetic resolution of this split, at integration (picture 3).

FIGURE 7.6   Picture 2.

5 Ethical issues: Artificial insemination raises various ethical issues, such as the use of donor sperm or eggs, the storage of embryos and the selection of certain characteristics of the child.
6 Psychological effects: The process of artificial insemination can be emotionally stressful and lead to stress, anxiety and depression. It is important that couples receive psychological support throughout the process.

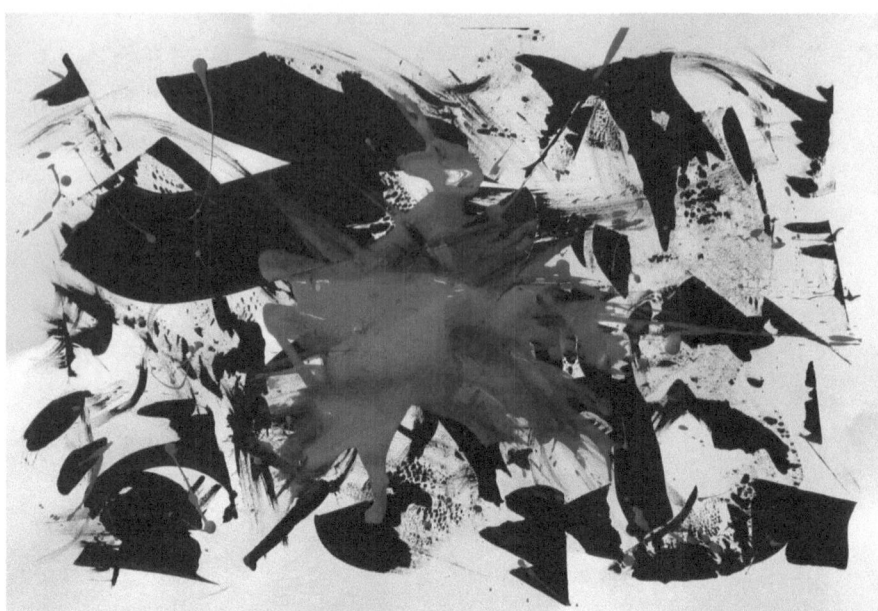

FIGURE 7.7 Picture 3.

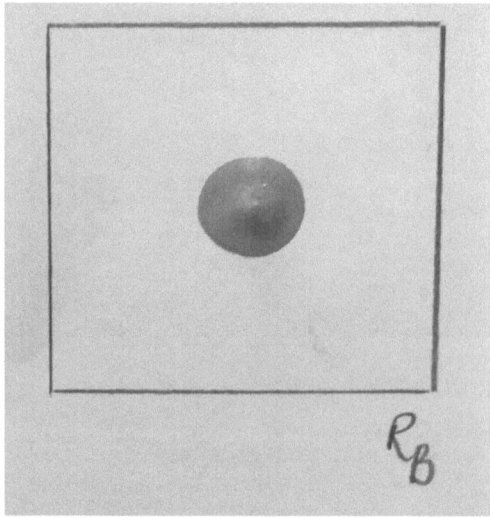

FIGURE 7.8 Picture 4. Painting of another cancer patient: The golden core. The self-confidence she developed after many years of art therapy in order to be able to deal with her primal pain (her mother's attempted abortion) and rediscover her primal resource (picture 4).

7 Long-term consequences for the child: Studies have shown that children born through artificial insemination generally do not have an increased risk of developmental problems or health problems. However, there is some evidence that certain ART procedures may be associated with a slightly increased risk of premature birth or low birth weight.

It is important to note that assisted reproduction is a complex area and individual circumstances and factors must be taken into account. Each case is unique, and it is advisable to consult professionals in the field of ART for specific information and advice (Auhagen-Stephanos 2017).

Summary

A good bond between people is the strongest resilience! Good bonds and relationships are the best protection against the dangers of life.

Prenatal attachment research, both quantitative and therapeutic, has impressively demonstrated the link between prenatal attachment qualities and mental health across the lifespan. These fundamental extensions of developmental theory and attachment theory represent a paradigm shift for medicine and psychology. Humanity is learning more and more about how all human life is shaped by attachment and relationship qualities from conception onwards and how much healing potential lies in these levels of enlightenment.

Ray Castellino, a leading prenatal psychologist, has formulated eight principles for conscious parenting:

Eight guiding principles for conscious parenting

Principle **1**: All behaviour is a communication. Behaviour reflects the internal state of the individual and the relationship's level of connection.

Principle **2**: The parent–child relationship is more important than any behavioural intervention, consequence or punishment.

Principle **3**: Children unfold neurosequentially, and quality, connected relationships allow for the unfolding. A need met will go away; a need unmet is here to stay.

Principle **4**: Behaviours occur on a continuum. Behaviours in children (and parents, too) correlate to the parents' own neurodevelopment and attachment status.

Principle **5**: Parental interpretation of behaviours comes from both a conscious and subconscious place, resulting in positive or negative neurophysiological feedback loops.

Principle **6**: All individuals have a right and a responsibility to learn to express their feelings appropriately. Feelings allow us to connect to our internal guidance system.

Principle **7**: Children need boundaries. We can set appropriate limits for our children while still respecting their needs and feelings – if we are aware of ourselves. (We can ask, for example, "Is this about me? Is this about them? Are my children communicating a need? Is the boundary I'm setting necessary, or is this an opportunity for me to grow?")

Principle **8**: No man is an island. We need to create communities of support for ourselves and for our children. We need to take care of ourselves so that we can take care of our children.

Literature

Ammaniti M, Gallese V (2014) *The birth of intersubjectivity. Psychodynamics, neurobiology and the self.* W. W. Norton & Company, New York.

Auhagen-Stephanos U (2017) *The mother-embryo dialogue. Fertility and infertility in the mirror of psychotherapy.* Psychosozial, Gießen.

Bretherton I (1992) "The origins of attachment theory: John Bowlby and Mary Ainsworth". In: *Developmental Psychology* 28: 759–775. https://doi.org/10.1037/0012-1649.28.5.759

Brandon A (2009) "A history of the theory of prenatal attachment". In: *Journal of Prenatal Perinatal Psychology Health* Summer; 23(4): 201–222.

Centers for Disease Control and Prevention (2021, July 27). Breastfeeding benefits both baby and mom. Centers for Disease Control and Prevention. Retrieved January 1, 2023, from https://www.cdc.gov/nccdphp/dnpao/features/breastfeeding-benefits/index.html

Chamberlain D (1988) *Babies remember birth.* Jeremy P. Tarcher, Los Angeles.

Condon JT (1993) "The assessment of antenatal emotional attachment: Development of a questionnaire instrument". In: *British Journal of Medical Psychology* 66: 167–183.

Conley, O. (2010). Birth without Violence (1975), by Frederick, The Embryo Project Encyclopedia. https://embryo.asu.edu/pages/birth-without-violence-1975-frederick-leboyer

Cranley MS (1981) "Development of a tool for the measurement of maternal attachment during pregnancy". In: *Nursing Research* 30: 281–284.

Evertz K (2020) "The inner child or the "inner child"? Confusion during pregnancy and its lifelong consequences". In: Gouni O et al. (eds.) *Change – Birthing & parenting at times of crisis.* Cosmoanelixis, Athens, 2021, 293–334.

Evertz K (2021a) "A visual exploration of psychodynamics in problematic pregnancies: Case studies in analytic-aesthetic art therapy". In: Evertz K et al. (eds.) *Handbook for prenatal psychology – Integrating research and practice.* Springer, Heidelberg, New York, 309–331.

Evertz K (2021b) "The prenatal dimension: Images in art and therapy". In: Evertz K et al. (eds.) *Handbook for prenatal psychology - Integrating research and practice.* Springer Nature, Cham, New York, 713–751.

Evertz K (2022) "Die Welt neu spüren – Die transgenerational-systemisch und pränatal fundierte methodenintegrative Psychotherapie – Integrative Kunst- und Körpertherapie". In: Klippel-Heidekrüger M, Janus L (eds.) *Diverse approaches to pre-linguistic and natal experience.* Mattes Verlag, Heidelberg, 271–292.

Evertz K, Janus L, Linder R (2021) *Handbook of prenatal and perinatal psychology – Integrating research and practice*. Springer Nature, Heidelberg, New York.

Fonagy P, Steele H, Steele M (1991) "Maternal representations of attachment during pregnancy predict the organisation of infant-mother attachment at one year of age". In: *Child Development* 62: 891–905.

Goertz-Schroth A, Schroth G, Phillips R (2023) "Prenatal bonding (BA) as a breakthrough in improving pregnancy, birth, and postpartum outcomes". In: *Journal for Prenatal and Perinatal Psychology and Health* 37(1): 1–21.

Hesketh T, Lu L, Xing ZW (2011) "The consequences of son preference and sex-selective abortion in China and other Asian countries". In: *CMAJ* 2011 September 6; 183(12): 1374–1377. https://doi.org/10.1503/cmaj.101368

Hidas G, Raffai J (2006) *Umbilical cord of the soul*. Psychosozial, Giessen.

Huttunen MO, Niskanen P (1978) "Prenatal loss of father and psychiatric disorders". In: *Archives of General Psychiatric* 35(4): 429–431.

Janus L (2000) *The psychoanalysis of the prenatal period and birth*. Psychosozial, Gießen.

Janus L, Evertz K (2008). *Kunst als kulturelles Bewusstsein geburtlicher und vorgeburtlicher Erfahrungen*. Mattes, Heidelberg.

Janus L (2021) "The history of prenatal psychology". In: Evertz K et al. (eds.) *Handbook of prenatal psychology*. Springer, New York, 3–8.

Jeličić, L., Veselinović, A., Ćirović, M., Jakovljević, V., Raičević, S., & Subotić, M. (2022). Maternal distress during pregnancy and the postpartum period: Underlying mechanisms and child's developmental outcomes - a narrative review. *International Journal of Molecular Sciences*, 23(22), 13932. https://doi.org/10.3390/ijms232213932

Kennell, J., Klaus, M., McGrath, S., Robertson, S., & Hinkley, C. (1991). Continuous emotional support during labor in a US hospital: A randomized controlled trial. *Journal of the American Medical Association*, 2665 (17), 2197–2201.

Koch J (2012) "Das Leben vor der Geburt". In: Der Spiegel, No. 25/18 June 2012, 120–128.

Linder R (2021) "Love, pregnancy, conflict, and solution: On the way to an understanding of conflicted pregnancy". In: Evertz K et al. (eds.) *Handbook for prenatal psychology – Integrating research and practice*. Springer Nature, Cham, New York, 337–346.

Lindgren K (2001) "Relationships among maternal-fetal attachment, prenatal depression, and health practices in pregnancy". In: *Research in Nursing & Health* 24: 203–217.

Lumley J (1982) "Attitudes to the foetus among primigravidae". In: *Journal of Paediatrics and Child Health* 18(2): 106–109.

Mikhail MS, Freda MC, Merkatz RB, Polizzotto R, Mazloom E, Merkatz IR (1991) "The effect of fetal movement counting on maternal attachment to fetus". In: *American Journal of Obstetrics & Gynecology* 165(4 Pt 1): 988–991.

Molenaar NM, Tiemeier H, van Rossum EFC, Hillegers MHJ, Bockting CLH, Hoogendijk WJG, van den Akker EL, Lambregtse-van den Berg MP, El Marroun H (2019) "Prenatal maternal psychopathology and stress and offspring HPA axis function at 6 years". In: *Psychoneuroendocrinology*, 99, 120–127. https://doi.org/10.1016/j.psyneuen.2018.09.003

Moncher FJ (1996) "The relationship of maternal adult attachment style and risk of physical child abuse". In: *Journal of Interpersonal Violence* 11(3): 335–350.

Monk C, Feng T, Lee S, Krupska I, Champagne FA, Tycko B (2016) "Distress during pregnancy: Epigenetic regulation of placenta glucocorticoid-related genes and fetal neurobehaviour". In: *American Journal of Psychiatry* 173(7): 705–713.

Müller A (2020) *Zusammenfassungde interne Auswertungen der Beratungsstelle zum Thema Schwangerschaftsabbruch.* Counselling centre: Schwanger – Du bist nicht allein e.V., Berlin, unpublished.

Phillips R (2012) Changing the practice of skin-to-skin contact in the first hour after birth to increase breastfeeding rates. In: *Platform Presentation, 17th Annual Conference of the Academy of Breastfeeding Medicine*, Chicago, IL.

Phillips R (2013). "The sacred hour: Uninterrupted skin-to-skin contact immediately after birth". *Newborn and Infant Nursing Reviews*, 13(2): 67–72.

Pollock PH, Percy A (1999) "Maternal antenatal attachment style and potential fetal abuse". In: *Child Abuse & Neglect* 23(12): 1345–1357.

Priel B, Besser A (2000) "Adult attachment styles, early relationships, antenatal attachment, and perceptions of infant temperament: A study of first-time mothers". In: *Personal Relationships* 7(3): 291–310.

Raffai J (2014) "Effects of parental conflicts in the intrauterine space". In: Evertz K, Janus L, Linder R (eds.) *Lehrbuch der Pränatalen Psychologie*. Mattes, Heidelberg, 556–570.

Raffai J (2021) "The impact of parental conflict in the intrauterine realm". In: Evertz K, Janus L, Linder R (eds.) *Handbook of prenatal and perinatal psychology*. Springer Nature, Cham, New York, 599–610.

Shreffler KM, Spierling TN, Jespersen JE, Tiemeyer S (2021) "Pregnancy Intendedness, Maternal-Fetal Bonding, and Postnatal Maternal-Infant Bonding". In: *Infant Mental Health Journal* 2021 May, 42(3): 362–373. doi:10.1002/imhj.21919.

Simons SSH, Zijlmans MAC, Cillessen AHN, de Weerth C (2019) Maternal prenatal and early postnatal distress and child stress responses at age 6. In: *Stress (Amsterdam, Netherlands)*, 22(6), 654–663. https://doi.org/10.1080/10253890.2019.1608945

UNFPA (2019). Trends in maternal mortality 2000 to 2017: Estimates by WHO, UNICEF, UNFPA, World Bank Group and the United Nations Population Division. Geneva: World Health Organization; 2019. License: CC BY-NC-SA 3.0 IGO. ISBN: 978-02-4-151648-8. https://www.unfpa.org/featured-publication/trends- maternal-mortality-2000-2017

UNICEF. (2023). https://www.un.org/sustainabledevelopment/decade-of-action/; https://www.unicef.org/health/maternal-newborn-and-child-survival, downloaded Jan 2023.

Van den Bergh, B. R. H., van den Heuvel, M. I., Lahti, M., Braeken, M., de Rooij, S. R., Entringer, S., Hoyer, D., Roseboom, T., Räikkönen, K., King, S., & Schwab, M. (2020). "Prenatal developmental origins of behavior and mental health: The influence of maternal stress in pregnancy". In: *Neuroscience and Biobehavioral Reviews* 117: 26–64. https://doi.org/10.1016/j.neubiorev.2017.07.003

Verny T, Kelly J (1981) *The secret life of the unborn child*. Summit Books, New York.

Weatherbee B (2024) "Distinct pathways drive anterior hypoblast specification in the implanting human embryo". In: *Nature Cell Biology* 26 (March 2024): 353–365.

Wu Y, Espinosa KM, Barnett SD, Kapse A, Quistorff JL, Lopez C, Andescavage N, Pradhan S, Lu YC, Kapse K, Henderson D, Vezina G, Wessel D, du Plessis AJ, Limperopoulos C (2022). Association of elevated maternal psychological distress, altered fetal brain, and offspring cognitive and social- emotional outcomes at 18 months. In: *Journal of the American Medical Association, Network Open*, 5(4): e229244. https://doi.org/10.1001/jamanetworkopen.2022.9244.

8

CLINICAL IMPLICATIONS

Psychosocial interventions during pregnancy

Pregnancy is a time of fundamental emotional and physical changes for mother and child and also for the father. The maturing process of becoming father and mother, when previously you were "only" lovers, also takes place in the positive and sometimes negative moods and tensions but sometimes also in physical symptoms. A pregnancy also affects the prenatal and birth history of the father and mother. Prenatal psychology utilises this knowledge in the psychosocial support of pregnant couples and in crisis interventions to support necessary medical interventions.

The most recent results of the Pforzheim study, for example, show a significant reduction in premature births from 8.8% to 2.2% among mothers who were treated with psychotherapy and social support (Linder 2024).

This chapter deals with the differentiation between physical and psychological stress and illnesses during pregnancy and the range of psychosocial support and treatments available. It also deals with the possibilities of prenatal counselling for parents-to-be and preventive measures to promote healthy prenatal development.

Psychosocial counselling for pregnant women, couples and families covers a broad spectrum. From body and movement work, yoga and relaxation techniques, mindfulness training and nutritional counselling, art therapy, birth preparation courses and breathing techniques, to psychosocial counselling and support in material or psychosocial emergencies for pregnant women, couples and family systems, to attachment analysis and psychotherapy and family therapy during pregnancy, there is a broad field of support, prevention and assistance. In a European comparison, the offers and services of the healthcare systems are very different. However, there has been a significant

DOI: 10.4324/9781003480242-8

increase in options over the last 20 years, as the importance of the topic for general health policy has been increasingly recognised.

Studies worldwide show that pregnant women suffer from moderate to high levels of stress (Woods et al. 2010). The need is therefore clear. Women have to fulfil many social, psychological and physical adaptation and developmental tasks.

Psychosocial interventions during pregnancy – an overview

There are a large number of studies that deal with psychosocial interventions during pregnancy. Some of the most important studies on this topic are:

1 A study by Vieten and Astin (2008) "Effects of a mindfulness-based intervention during pregnancy on prenatal stress and mood: results of a pilot study" showed that mindfulness-based interventions significantly reduce anxiety and negative effects during pregnancy (Vieten & Astin 2008).
2 A study by Field et al. (1999) investigated the effects of massage therapy on the mental well-being of pregnant women. The results showed that regular massage during pregnancy led to a reduction in anxiety and depression (Field et al. 1999).
3 A meta-analysis by Dennis et al. (2007) investigated the effectiveness of group interventions for the prevention of pregnancy depression. The results showed that group interventions can help to reduce the risk of pregnancy depression (Dennis et al. 2007).
4 Studies by Grote et al. (Grote & Bledsoe 2006; Grote et al. 2015) investigated the effects of cognitive behavioural therapy on the psychological well-being of pregnant women with anxiety disorders. The results showed that the therapy helped to reduce anxiety symptoms and improve psychological well-being (Grote & Bledsoe 2006; Grote et al. 2015).
5 A study by Goertz-Schroth (Goertz-Schroth et al.2023) investigated the effects of attachment analysis during pregnancy. It showed a significant reduction in pregnancy and labour complications. Attachment analysis supports communication between mother and child on sensory, emotional and language levels.

These studies show that psychosocial interventions in pregnancy are effective in promoting the psychological well-being of pregnant women and reducing potential negative effects on maternal and infant health. It is important to conduct further research in this area to better understand the effectiveness of different interventions and to promote their implementation in clinical practice.

Other noteworthy studies:

– Mindfulness-Based Methods and Meditation (Pan et al. 2019; Vieten & Astin 2008; Frederiksen et al. 2017),

- Yoga (Chen et al. 2017; Narendran et al. 2005),
- Mind-Body Interventions (Beddoe & Lee 2008; Marc et al. 2011),
- Music (Shimada et al. 2020, Chang et al. 2015; van Willenswaard et al. 2017),
- Hypnosis (Legrand et al. 2017; Catsaros & Wendland 2020),
- Nutrition (Gluckman et al. 2015),
- Physical Activity (Dietz et al. 2016),
- Positive Psychological Intervention (Matvienko-Sikar & Dockray 2016),
- Mindfulness-Based Cognitive Therapy (MBCT) (Tomfohr-Madsen et al. 2016),
- Cognitive Behavioural Therapy (Frederiksen et al. 2015),
- Cognitive Behavioural Stress Management (CBSM) (Urizar 2023),
- Psychoeducation (Beddoe & Lee 2008).

General preventive measures to promote healthy prenatal development

1 Healthy diet: A balanced and nutritious diet during pregnancy is crucial for the healthy development of the foetus. It is important to ensure an adequate intake of vitamins, minerals and omega-3 fatty acids.
2 Avoidance of harmful substances: Pregnant women should avoid the consumption of alcohol, tobacco and illegal drugs, as these substances can increase the risk of complications and developmental disorders.
3 Regular prenatal care: Regular visits to a doctor, midwife and attachment counsellor are important to monitor the health of mother and child and to strengthen and support the bond between mother and child. This enables early detection of problems and appropriate medical care and psychological support.
4 Attachment analysis (prenatal bonding) to strengthen and build the emotional relationship between mother and child.
5 Stress management: Pregnant women should learn and practise stress management techniques, as high levels of stress can increase the risk of complications. Relaxation techniques such as meditation, yoga or breathing exercises can be helpful.
6 Sufficient exercise: Moderate physical activity during pregnancy can improve blood circulation, boost metabolism and promote general well-being. However, it is important to consult your doctor and pay attention to your body's individual needs.
7 Sleep hygiene: Adequate sleep is important for the health of both mother and child. Pregnant women should ensure good sleep hygiene by creating a comfortable sleeping environment, maintaining regular bedtimes and practising relaxation techniques before going to bed.
8 Avoiding infections: Pregnant women should take measures to minimise the risk of infection. These include regular hand washing, immunisation according to the doctor's recommendations and avoiding contact with infectious people or places.

9 Social network support: A strong social network can help pregnant women reduce stress and receive emotional support. It is important to surround yourself with family, friends or a supportive community.
10 Prenatal education: Learning about pregnancy, birth and caring for a newborn can help to reduce anxiety and increase confidence in your own ability as a parent. Prenatal education courses can be helpful. It is particularly important for parents to share their biographical and family backgrounds.
11 Early intervention for risk factors: If a pregnant woman has certain risk factors, such as a history of complications or genetic conditions, it is important to seek early medical and psychosocial counselling and care (Weintraub 1992; Verny 2003).

Clinical implications – psychosocial intervention options during pregnancy for mother, child and father

1 Miscarriage, stillbirth, premature birth
2 Pregnancy complications
3 Psychological problems during pregnancy – pregnancy ambivalences
4 Prenatal medical interventions
5 Prenatal trauma and birth trauma

Miscarriage, stillbirth, premature birth

A stillbirth is when there are no recognisable signs of life after the birth of a child and the child has a birth weight of over 500 grams; otherwise, it is referred to as a miscarriage. The diagnosis is intrauterine foetal death (IUFT) or infans mortuus. Perinatal mortality includes stillbirths and infants who die up to one week after birth. Infant mortality refers to deaths in the first year after birth.

The loss of a pregnancy or a child before birth triggers grief that needs to be overcome, regardless of the age of the pregnancy. As a rule, the more developed the child was, the greater the grief and pain. The experience of pain and the necessary grief work vary greatly from person to person, but prenatal psychology always assumes that the loss was traumatic.

In Germany, parents were not able to say goodbye to their child until the 1980s. The mother was sedated if a stillbirth was to be expected and the child was removed without being shown to her. Thanks to the advancing psychological knowledge of the necessity of mourning processes, it is now the norm worldwide for parents to be allowed to see their child one last time and to bury it while also receiving psychosocial support.

Some women or couples do not manage to develop new perspectives on life during their grief. Not infrequently, subsequent pregnancies are also characterised by anxiety. Those affected can be supported through conversations that give them space to articulate their feelings. Many of those affected also suffer from the fact that the loss of a child during pregnancy is often not recognised as an unfortunate experience, especially in the case of early terminations in the first trimester. Understanding friends, relatives or even staff at a pregnancy counselling centre can be helpful in coping with the grief. A persistently depressive reaction to the loss may require psychotherapeutic treatment.

In prenatal psychology, every child, even a child who died intrauterine or an aborted child, is counted as part of the family system. However, it is important that the severity of individual experiences is taken into account! It is not about moral judgements or ethical evaluations but about clarifying the feelings in the family system. It is important that every implanted child, as two-thirds of pregnancies end at implantation, indicates an energy and strength of affirmation of life in the couple's relationship or in the family system. The loss of a child often causes precisely the pain of not wanting life to go on. After all, it is a disappointment of a hopeful expectation that life can be passed on and, philosophically speaking, that one's own person will continue to live on in the child. Children are the only real transcendence! Even if the loss of a prenatal child is not so deeply considered and felt by every couple, these levels are unconsciously touched and often require empathic resonance. In addition, children who died in utero not only have an effect on the self-image of the mother and the couple but also on existing or subsequent siblings.

Therapeutic observation of the surrogate child syndrome is very important. Children who are conceived after a stillborn child often have the feeling that they are not fully recognised themselves, but that the parents' gaze is still focused on the deceased child. These children often feel restricted in their development because they feel they are not meant and as if their parents' love is still focussed on something else more valuable. Also, the mother's emotional caution or fear after the loss of a child often results in a tense attitude during the new pregnancy, so that another child is not lost.

Adult patients can "remember" their needy and sad mother very well, who was still suffering from the loss of a child when she was already pregnant with them.

Premature birth

The earliest premature birth to date is a boy from Alabama who was saved in an emergency operation at 21 weeks and one day with 420 grams. His twin sister died. As a rule, children born after 22–24 weeks can be saved today. Intensive medical measures and incubators and skin-to-skin contact with the parents (kangaroo method) are the elementary means of saving the child's life.

Kangaroo mother care (KMC) is recommended as routine care for all premature or low birth weight infants. KMC can be started in a health centre or at home and should be provided for 8–24 hours per day (as many hours as possible). There is a strong recommendation and high certainty of evidence (Linderkamp 2021a, 2021b; WHO 2022).

In addition to medical and nursing care, parents and child can receive psychosocial support. Prenatal psychology has been able to establish important standards in the care of premature babies, in particular by evaluating the importance of physical contact.

This skin-to-skin contact had surprising consequences for the parents and children: the children's brains developed better and their bodily functions matured more quickly. In the end, child and parents were much better bonded. The children had to be ventilated less and for shorter periods of time. The mother produced more milk and the child learnt to drink more quickly instead of being fed passively via a tube. The real breakthrough towards mother-child-centred care came with the WHO's Baby-Friedly Hospital Initiative in 1991.

(Linderkamp 2021, p. 148)

Prematurity can have long-term effects on life. Premature babies have an increased developmental risk and therefore require careful medical and psychosocial attention and support (Hüning & Jäkel 2021).

From a prenatal psychological perspective, the question is why the "co-operation" between mother and child is called into question: What emotional conditions from the mother's and father's history hinder the normal course of development? What systemic stress is causing the child to (have to) leave the mother earlier than planned? Preterm birth attempts can therefore also be influenced and even prevented by psychosocial or psychotherapeutic interventions (Goertz-Schroth 2023).

Stillbirth

Most stillbirths could be prevented with qualified healthcare and care during pregnancy.

According to the report "A Neglected Tragedy: The Global Burden of Stillbirths", 84 per cent of stillbirths occur in low- and middle-income countries. Germany is at 0.24 per cent, France at 0.39 per cent. The highest rates are in Nigeria with 4.2 per cent and Pakistan with 4.7 per cent. According to a United Nations report, it is estimated that there are almost 2 million stillbirths worldwide every year.

(Wikipedia 2024)

There is still a lack of sufficient resources worldwide, especially in poorer countries, to provide sufficient professional support and protection during pregnancy. This is also one of humanity's great peace projects.

Pregnancy complications

Pregnancy is first and foremost a unique, positive experience for parents-to-be. It usually runs smoothly and possible complications can be avoided by having regular check-ups throughout the nine months.

Even high-risk pregnancies (including expectant mothers over the age of 35, women who have already had a miscarriage, multiple pregnancies) usually go smoothly today, thanks to the medical possibilities.

Nevertheless, it can be useful to find out about possible complications. Ectopic pregnancy, miscarriage, neural tube defects, listeriosis and toxoplasmosis, for example, are the most common complications during pregnancy.

Pregnancy complications are unfavourable developments during pregnancy that can be potentially life-threatening for the foetus and mother. They arise either as a result of the pregnancy itself or due to pre-existing maternal conditions. The most common pregnancy complications include thromboembolic events, haemorrhage and hypertension.

In principle, pregnancy complications can originate from the mother, the foetus and/or the placenta. Some of the complications can occur at the same time or be mutually dependent.

The most common pregnancy complications and diseases

1 Early miscarriage: Pregnancy can lead to an early miscarriage in the first few weeks due to various factors, such as genetic abnormalities or hormonal imbalances.
2 Ectopic pregnancy: In an ectopic pregnancy, the fertilised egg implants outside the uterus, usually in the fallopian tubes. This can lead to serious complications and requires immediate medical treatment.
3 Gestational diabetes: Some women develop temporary diabetes during pregnancy, known as gestational diabetes. This can lead to complications for both mother and child and requires a special diet and possibly insulin treatment.
4 Pre-eclampsia: Pre-eclampsia is a serious condition characterised by high blood pressure and damage to organs such as the liver and kidneys. It usually occurs after the 20th week of pregnancy and requires close monitoring and possibly premature delivery (Linder 2021b).
5 Placental abruption: A placental abruption occurs when the placenta detaches prematurely from the uterine wall. This can lead to heavy bleeding and can be life-threatening for both the mother and the baby.

6 Complications of multiple pregnancies: With twins or other multiple pregnancies, there is an increased risk of complications such as premature birth, growth retardation or umbilical cord problems.

7 Malformations: Some babies can develop congenital malformations during pregnancy, which can range from mild to severe impairments. This can have genetic or environmental causes.

8 The most dangerous infections are:

Cytomegalovirus (CMV): An infection with CMV can lead to serious complications during pregnancy, such as malformations in the foetus, premature birth or neurological damage.

Rubella: Rubella infection during pregnancy can lead to severe congenital malformations in the foetus, such as deafness, heart defects or mental retardation.

Toxoplasmosis: Infection with toxoplasmosis during pregnancy can cause serious damage to the foetus, including inflammation of the brain, eye damage and mental retardation.

Listeriosis: A listeriosis infection during pregnancy can lead to a serious illness that can affect the foetus's central nervous system.

Syphilis: An untreated syphilis infection during pregnancy can lead to serious complications, such as premature birth, stillbirth or congenital syphilis in the newborn.

HIV/AIDS: Transmission of HIV from mother to child during pregnancy or at birth can lead to HIV infection in the newborn.

Hepatitis B: A hepatitis B infection during pregnancy can lead to a chronic infection in the newborn and increase the risk of liver disease.

Zika virus: Zika infection during pregnancy can lead to severe congenital malformations in the foetus, such as microcephaly (abnormally small head circumference) and neurological problems.

Chickenpox (varicella): A chickenpox infection during pregnancy can lead to serious complications in the foetus, such as skin lesions, eye damage or developmental delays.

Flu (influenza): A severe flu infection during pregnancy can lead to complications, such as premature birth, low birth weight or even death of the foetus (Rath & Baltzer 2005; Steller & Goerke 2018).

Prevention

Underlying maternal illnesses should be managed as well as possible. Close obstetric care and regular check-ups can minimise the risk for mother and child and enable early diagnosis of complications.

In the case of medical diagnoses during pregnancy, prenatal psychology significantly helps to achieve better healing results and preventive avoidance through psychosocial support and therapeutic treatment. Pregnancy complications always have a psychological background, but too little time and attention is often given to dealing with them (Evertz 2021; Goertz-Schroth et al. 2023; Linder 2021b).

For example, the dangerous disease of gestosis. In prenatal psychology, gestosis is always an expression of the mother's strong ambivalence: on the one hand, she feels more complete and fulfilled with the baby than ever before in her life, and all the more so the greater the experiences of loneliness and trauma-induced relationship disorders are. However, the closer the birth approaches, the more the unconscious fear of separation, detachment and loss grows, which triggers the old life-historical experiences of loss and loneliness. However, there is an unconscious desire for the pregnancy to end as quickly as possible because the tension between the desire to keep and the separation becomes too great and seems emotionally unresolvable. "Pregnancy poisoning" is an old term for gestosis and HELLP syndrome. Pregnancy is also emotionally "poisoned" by the life-historical injuries to the pregnant woman's femininity. As a rule, she was not sufficiently strengthened in her feminine identity in the family system because, for example, she was desired as a boy but not as a girl. This unbearable tension of now having to be a woman as a result of the pregnancy, but also feeling the lack of emotional support in her life history, is discharged in a whole-body defence against the pregnancy, which can now become life-threatening for mother and child in gestosis. Today, we can treat these syndromes well medically and provide good psychotherapeutic support. Gestosis usually ends in a caesarean birth a few weeks before the due date (Linder 2021b).

Mental health problems during pregnancy

Psychological problems such as mood instability are often triggered by hormones in the first trimester of pregnancy. Perhaps the pregnancy is burdened by financial or partnership problems, or perhaps it was unplanned and a termination of pregnancy was on the cards. Physical changes or a complicated pregnancy can also lead to psychological problems. Counselling support during pregnancy often helps. Psychological problems that occurred during pregnancy do not necessarily have to continue after the birth. However, you should be aware of them.

The most common psychological problems during pregnancy are

1 Pregnancy depression, denied or suppressed pregnancy
2 Pregnancy ambivalence and pregnancy conflict
3 Fear of the birth
4 Pregnancy fears

5 Sleep disorders
6 Eating disorders
7 Stress and overload, psychosocial strain
8 Relationship problems
9 Body image problems
10 Obsessive-compulsive disorders
11 Partnership violence
12 Disappointment about the gender of the child – gender disappointment
13 Twin loss
14 Unfulfilled desire to have children – infertility

Notes on the most common problems:

Depression during or after pregnancy/postpartum depression

Brooding, fear of failure, sleep disorders, frequent crying, irritability, emotional emptiness or feelings of guilt can be symptoms of a temporary low mood or also indicate depression, which can occur during or only after pregnancy. Those affected are often plagued by self-doubt and are seemingly unable to form an intimate bond with their child. Unfortunately, a lack of understanding from those around them and shame often mean that help is only sought at a late stage.

Postpartum depression can occur at any time in the first two years after giving birth. According to an attachment analysis, postpartum depression does not occur, which once again shows how important the prenatal relationship is

It still occurs in around 10–15% of all women after childbirth, 75% of them after the first birth. Fathers can also be affected, albeit less frequently. The causes and risk factors for its occurrence can be varied. These include a history of mental illness in oneself or in the family, depressive episodes during pregnancy, a conflict-ridden pregnancy, e.g. due to problems in the partnership or family, inadequate support from the environment and one's own high expectations of being a perfect mother. It is not always possible to organise and control life with a baby according to one's own ideas and this causes strong women in particular to question their competence. The hormonal changes after the birth obviously play a lesser role.

This can take different forms, from changing moods to serious suicidal thoughts. The duration depends on the severity of the illness and can last several weeks or months, rarely even longer.

If more severe depression develops, psychotherapeutic or psychiatric outpatient or inpatient treatment (ideally in a mother and child centre) is necessary. Prescribing medication may also be helpful when weighing up the risks and benefits during pregnancy and while breastfeeding.

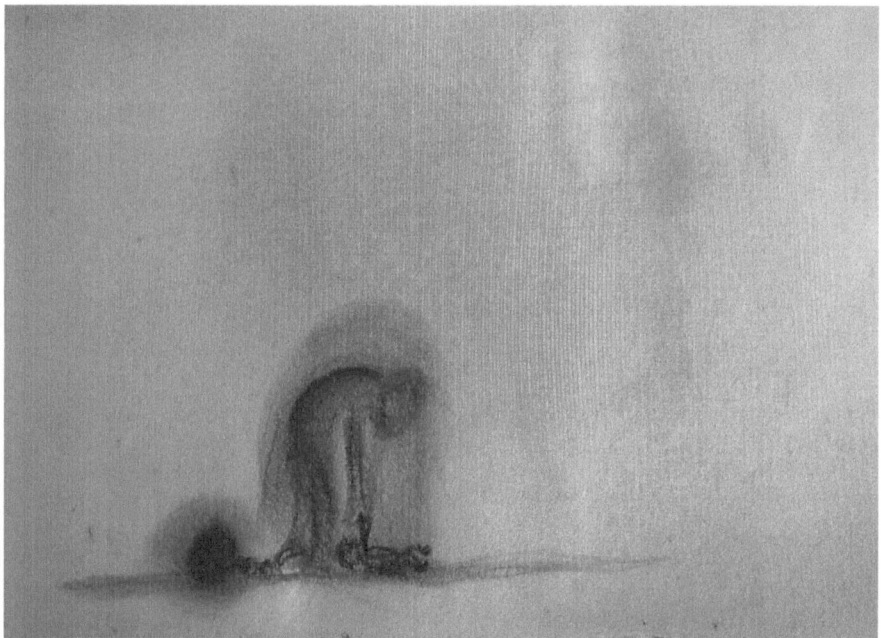

FIGURE 8.1 Drawing by a depressed patient about her pregnant mother.

There is a certain risk of recurrence, but this does not mean that further pregnancies should be avoided. Early psychosocial counselling can be helpful here.

Social support for the mother in everyday life from her partner, family or good friends can be a preventative measure (Figure 8.1).

Postpartum psychosis At around 0.2%, this occurs much less frequently during pregnancy or after childbirth. The most important risk factors or triggers here are also mental disorders in the past or in the family, the birth experience and the hormonal changes. The onset is usually quite acute with symptoms such as concentration and thought disorders, impulsivity, agitation, conspicuous behaviour, irritability, depression, aggression, restlessness, anxiety disorders, obsessive thoughts, delusions, hallucinations, disturbed sleep patterns and suicidal thoughts. Psychiatric, usually inpatient, treatment is essential and depends on the symptoms. As a rule, drug therapy is also necessary and possible.

(Pro Familia 2024)

From a prenatal psychological perspective, maternal depression during pregnancy is usually also an attempt by the mother to come to terms with her own troubled childhood, birth or pregnancy experience, irrespective of current

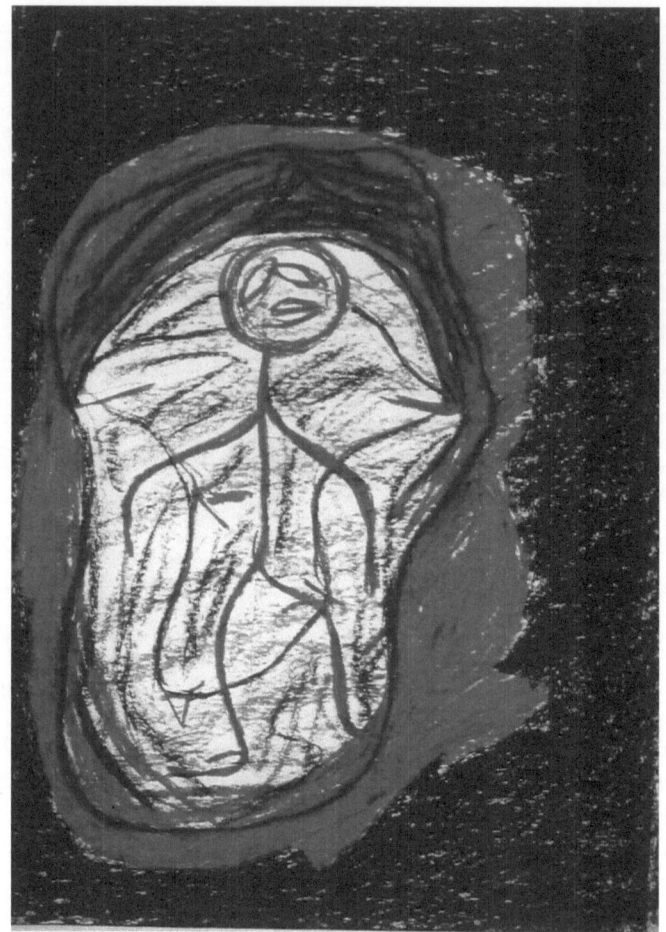

FIGURE 8.2 "Starved child", the emotional deficiency becomes clear in many art therapy images if the mother was suffering from depression during pregnancy.

conflicts and problems. The current pregnancy is always a strong trigger for the woman's own unresolved traumas and stressful life experiences (Figure 8.2). For many women, these life-historical burdens also lead to the decision not to have children, which, on the one hand, leaves sadness but, on the other hand, can be very responsible. However, women who have become pregnant only learn during pregnancy that expecting a child can also be very stressful and often do not know what the reason for "bad feelings" is (Schroth 2021).

Repressed or denied pregnancy

There are women who carry painful experiences from their past that have not been dealt with. When these women become pregnant, repressed and denied pregnancies can occur, sometimes with extreme psychological repression. In one case of a repressed pregnancy, the woman actually believes that she is not pregnant and interprets her body changes as weight gain or illness, for example, sometimes even until the birth. In the case of pregnancy denial, the woman knows that she is pregnant but does everything she can to prevent the world around her from finding out.

Typical characteristics of such cases are:

- Reduced intelligence
- Acute experiences of separation
- Chronic family or interpersonal conflicts
- Chronic eating disorders
- Severe mental disorder
- Autonomy endeavours
- Indifferent or listless relationship to sexuality
- Misinterpretation of pregnancy signs

(Wessel et al. 2002)

Gender disappointment

Gender disappointment, also known as gender disappointment syndrome or gender disappointment disorder, refers to the feeling of sadness, frustration or dissatisfaction that some people experience when the gender of their baby does not match their expectations or desires. It is important to note that gender disappointment is not yet recognised as a clinical diagnosis in the Diagnostic and Statistical Manual of Mental Disorders (DSM-5).

From a prenatal psychological perspective, disappointment about the child's gender, especially if it is emotionally intense, often means a future weakening of the child's sexual identity. This aspect is given too little consideration today when it comes to the gender insecurities of adolescents, although it could be very supportive. Whenever hidden and suppressed feelings are held back in family systems out of shame, this makes it more difficult to find a personal identity, including sexual identity.

See also Chapter 7 on "Sex-selective abortion".

Twin pregnancies

The two best-known forms of twin formation are:

Identical twins (*monozygotic*)

The fertilised egg cell (zygote) divides in the course of development, the cells resulting from the division also divide and so on. If a division into two cell populations occurs at a very early stage of development, two embryonic systems can develop. Both are then *monozygotic* from a single fertilised egg cell with the same *genetic material* and therefore the same *genetic make-up*. Depending on the time of separation, twin forms with separate or common *egg membranes of chorion or amnion* develop.

Fraternal twins (*dizygotic*)

Within one cycle, two eggs have matured and each has been fertilised by a different *sperm*. The two zygotes give rise to *dizygotic* twins with different genetic material and their own chorion and amnion.

What research results are available on the subject of twin loss?

The loss of twins during pregnancy or after birth is a tragic event that can be emotionally distressing. There is limited research on this topic, but here are some important research findings:

1 Frequency: The frequency of twin loss varies depending on the study and population group. A study from 2018 found that the rate of twin loss is around 3–4% of all pregnancies.
2 Causes: The causes of twin loss can be varied and range from genetic abnormalities and complications during pregnancy to unexplained factors. Some studies have shown that certain risk factors such as advanced maternal age, multiple pregnancies or previous miscarriages can increase the risk of twin loss.
3 Impact on parents: The loss of twins can have a significant impact on the mental health and well-being of parents. Studies have shown that parents who experience twin loss may have an increased risk of grief, depression, anxiety and post-traumatic stress disorder.
4 Long-term effects: There is limited research on the long-term effects of twin loss on parents and their families. However, some studies have shown that parents who experience twin loss may face long-term feelings of grief and loss. There may also be an impact on the parents' relationship with each other and on their future family planning decisions.

It is important to note that each twin loss is unique and that the individual experiences and reactions of the affected parents may vary. Twin loss can also be a particular issue in baby therapy, child and adolescent psychotherapy and adult therapy if the surviving child suffers attachment and relationship difficulties later in life as a result of the loss of the twin (Dilcher 2021).

Pregnancy conflict counselling

Finding out about a pregnancy can trigger contradictory feelings in women, men and couples, such as joy, but also uncertainty, fear or rejection.

If the woman and the man, or one of them, have very strong resistance to carrying the pregnancy to term, a psychosocial or psychotherapeutic assessment is always worthwhile.

There are counselling centres that offer support to pregnant couples in this situation. The counselling

- Enables you to address your thoughts, feelings and questions
- Can help them weigh up the pros and cons of carrying the pregnancy to term
- Accompanies you in your decision-making process with an open mind
- Provides them with information on financial and social assistance as well as legal rights before and after the birth of a child
- Informs you about the emotional and medical aspects, the legal basis and the cost of an abortion.

Counselling should be sensitive, respectful and open-ended and also include an offer for the time after the decision.

Contradictory feelings can cause stress after an abortion. These are often perceived differently by women and men. In these cases, individual or couples counselling can help to reorganise the life situation.

Abortions can have psychological consequences if it has not been clarified who is actually meant by the abortion of the child: the real child or the traumatised "inner child" of the mother or father. In addition to all the feelings that it is not right now, that there is no money, that it is not the right man, that the mother is generally in a bad way, the deeper biographical background in the clarification is often relieving (Evertz 2016, 2021, 2022).

See also Chapters 6, 7 and 9.

Pregnancy and experience of violence

Even if it would be more than desirable otherwise, women repeatedly become pregnant after physical or sexual violence or under psychological pressure. Or they experience violence and pressure during their pregnancy.

Preventing or minimising partner violence against
women during pregnancy

Violence against pregnant women by their partners is an important public health issue. It can cause physical and emotional harm to women, cause complications in pregnancy and damage the health of the child. It is unclear what type of intervention is best suited to protect women and their children during pregnancy and postpartum. Interventions that may work include counselling and psychotherapy to boost women's confidence and encourage them to develop strategies to avoid abuse. Referrals to social workers, mother and child centres or other community-based services can also help. Violent partners can be admitted to specialised therapy programmes.

Unfulfilled desire to have children

The longed-for pregnancy does not always materialise. The unfulfilled desire to have children becomes an emotional burden.

The causes of limited fertility or involuntary childlessness are very diverse. At a certain point, the question may arise as to whether medical help should be sought. However, you may also be undergoing reproductive medical treatment without having become pregnant. How long should the treatment be continued? Do you have to say goodbye to the desire to have your own child? What alternatives are there?

"When the Soul Says No" by Auhagen-Stephanos is a very good book on these questions. From a prenatal psychological point of view, the symptom of infertility often harbours family systemic traumas that have not yet been dealt with and which result in unconscious prohibitions against passing on life (Auhagen-Stephanos 2002, 2017; Evertz 2021).

Prenatal medical interventions – foetal surgery

There is rarely a need for surgery during pregnancy for diseases of the mother or the child. Operations on the mother are always a prenatal trauma for the child.

Foetal surgery refers to the possibility of prenatal surgery as part of in utero treatment for severe or life-threatening malformations or diseases of the growing foetus.

In 1981, the first operation was performed on a foetus, in which the mother's abdomen was opened and the foetus could be operated on, or even the foetus was removed for surgery. As a rule, the operations were and still are for spina bifida. Today, operations on the foetus can sometimes also be performed using minimally invasive techniques.

Examinations, indications and operable malformations

- Forms of spina bifida aperta
- Congenital diaphragmatic hernia
- Amniotic band syndrome
- Coccyx teratoma with heart failure
- Discordant twin pregnancies
- Acranius acardius
- Twin transfusion syndrome/fetofetal transfusion syndrome
- Congenital complete heart block, atrioventricular block (AV block) with heart failure

- Severe narrowing of the foetal aortic and pulmonary valve
- Supraventricular tachycardia = rapid heartbeat with heart failure
- Laryngeal and tracheal obstructions (foetal CHAOS, e.g. in laryngeal atresia)
- Foetal biopsies and diagnostic fetoscopies
- Gastroschisis
- Severe narrowing of the foramen ovale (foramen ovale restriction)
- Hydrothorax
- Posterior urethral valves (urinary outflow obstruction)
- Aortic isthmus stenosis (or interrupted aortic arch, underdevelopment of the left heart, left ventricular hypoplasia, coarctation)
- for premature rupture of the membranes (therapy to improve lung development)
  (German Centre for Fetal Surgery and Minimally Invasive Therapy (DZFT) 2024)

Traumatic birth

Many women, but also men, experience an unexpectedly stressful or even traumatic birth. An unplanned caesarean section, complications during the birth or even a life-threatening situation for mother or child, insensitive or inadequate care in the hospital and exceptionally strong contractions can have a lasting impact on the birth experience.

Even years after a difficult birth, the memory of the experience can still be unbearable. Self-doubt, attachment disorders, feelings of guilt and even depression and post-traumatic stress disorder are possible as a result. It is not uncommon for relationships and sexuality to suffer. The exchange with other mothers is avoided. Further pregnancies are avoided or the prospect of another birth is extremely anxiety-ridden.

Those affected need space and understanding to process their experiences and integrate them into their lives.

Clarifying, informative psychosocial counselling sessions can provide relief. If the disorder persists, psychotherapeutic treatment is recommended.

WHO recommendations for normal birth

In principle, these recommendations are based on this assumption,

1 That every woman has a fundamental right to comprehensive care during pregnancy.
2 That she is at the centre of all aspects of this care and participates in the planning, implementation and assessment of preventive measures.
3 That in addition to medical care, social, emotional and psychological factors are decisive for comprehensive care during pregnancy.

(WHO Intrapartum Care for a Positive Childbirth Experience 2018)

16 Recommendations of the World Health Organisation (WHO)
    Birth is not a disease

1 The entire public should be informed about the different methods of obstetric care so that every woman is able to find the method of obstetric care that is right for her.
2 The training of midwives and all professional groups who care for women and children during labour must be promoted. The care of a normal pregnancy, during labour and in the postpartum period is part of the remit of midwives and related professions.
3 All hospitals should make information about the obstetric care they provide (e.g. their caesarean section rate) freely available to pregnant women.
4 There is no justification whatsoever for a caesarean section rate above 10–15%.
5 A caesarean section once does not necessarily mean a caesarean section for all subsequent births. After such an operation, in which the uterus has been opened at a low-lying point, a vaginal delivery can be attempted if an intervention can be carried out quickly in an emergency.
6 There is no evidence that routine continuous electronic monitoring of the baby's heartbeat has a positive effect on the outcome of the birth.
7 There is no need to shave your pubic hair or have an enema before the birth.
8 During labour, pregnant women should not lie on their backs. They should be encouraged to walk around during labour and decide freely in which position they want to give birth.
9 Routine episiotomies are not justifiable.
10 Labour inductions should not take place out of convenience. Contraceptives should only be administered after strict medical indications.
11 Analgesic and anaesthetic drugs should not be used routinely but only to treat or prevent a complication during labour.
12 There is no scientific justification for the early opening of the amniotic sac as a routine procedure.
13 A healthy newborn belongs with its mother if the condition of both allows it. Observation of the child does not justify separation from the mother.
14 After the birth, the mother should be given the opportunity to breastfeed as soon as possible.
15 Obstetric facilities that take a critical approach to the use of technology and emphasise emotional, psychological and social aspects should be publicised. These projects should be promoted in order to serve as models for other obstetric facilities and to change public attitudes towards obstetrics.

16 Governments should consider creating regulations that allow the use of new birth technologies only after appropriate testing.

(The World Health Organization (WHO), Regional Office for Europe (EURO), Centre of Information on Public Health in the European Region (CIPHER))
    The most common birth traumas are:

1   Birth injuries: These include tears or cuts in the birth canal that can occur during labour and can lead to pain and complications.
2   Caesarean section: A caesarean section is a surgical procedure in which the baby is removed through an incision in the mother's abdomen. This can lead to physical and emotional trauma.
3   Premature birth: A premature birth occurs when the baby is born before the 37th week of pregnancy. Premature babies often have health problems and can spend a long time in hospital, which can lead to traumatisation.
4   Emergency caesarean section: An emergency caesarean section is an urgent surgical procedure that is performed if complications arise during labour. This can be very traumatic for the mother and the baby.
5   Birth complications: These include problems such as umbilical cord entanglement, shoulder dystocia (when the baby's shoulders get stuck in the birth canal) or placental abruption (when the placenta separates prematurely from the uterus). These complications can lead to injury or stress for mother and child.
6   Miscarriage: A miscarriage is the loss of a pregnancy before the 20th week. This can be very traumatic for the parents and lead to emotional and psychological stress.
7   Obstructed labour: Obstructed labour occurs when labour does not progress or the baby gets stuck in the birth canal. This can lead to a longer and more difficult labour and can be traumatic for both the mother and the baby.
8   Birth trauma due to medical interventions: Sometimes medical interventions such as the use of a suction cup or forceps during labour can lead to injury or trauma.
9   Postnatal depression: Postnatal depression is a form of depression that can occur after birth. It can impair the bond between mother and child and lead to emotional traumatisation.
10 Lack of support during labour: If a woman does not receive adequate support during labour, this can lead to a feeling of helplessness and trauma.

The application of prenatal psychological knowledge and corresponding methods can significantly reduce pregnancy and birth complications

(Goertz-Schroth 2023). The consequences of obstetric interventions are also well understood today (Emerson 2021).

(See Chapter 9).

Summary

The worldwide improvement in pregnancy and birth culture with a significant reduction in pregnancy complications, premature births and stillbirths still contrasts with a lack of information and a lack of social, psychological and medical options in many emerging and developing countries. This chapter summarises the possibilities of preventive measures for prenatal counselling, support and assistance for expectant parents.

In the industrialised nations, it is primarily a question of stepping up efforts to integrate psychosocial models alongside medical strategies in pregnancy support, obstetrics and neonatology.

Prenatal psychology can significantly increase the depth of understanding of all pregnancy and birth complications and serve as a background for all psychosocial services.

Therefore, we suggest that a better understanding of prenatal psychology can be an effective tool for the prediction and prevention of pregnancy complications and for personalised therapeutic interventions. In addition, consideration of the principles of prenatal psychology can support the development of skills among healthcare professionals. At a local and regional level, the networking of health and social workers can help to effectively prevent mental health complications and other diseases of our time.

(Linder 2021a, 2024)

Literature

Auhagen-Stephanos U (2002) *When the soul says no*. Kösel, Munich.

Auhagen-Stephanos U (2017) *The mother-embryo dialogue. Fertility and infertility in the mirror of psychotherapy*. Psychosozial, Gießen.

Beddoe AE, Lee KA (2008) "Mind-body interventions during pregnancy". In: *Journal of Obstetric, Gynecologic, & Neonatal Nursing* 37(2): 165–175. doi: 10.1111/j.1552-6909.2008.00218.x

Caritas (2024) https://www.caritas-koeln.de/hilfe-beratung/kinder-jugend-familie/ueberblick/

Catsaros S, Wendland J (2020) "Hypnosis-based interventions during pregnancy and childbirth and their impact on women's childbirth experience: A systematic review". In: *Midwifery*. 84: 102666. doi: 10.1016/j.midw.2020.102666.

Chang HC, Yu CH, Chen SY, Chen CH. (2015) "The effects of music listening on psychosocial stress and maternal-fetal attachment during pregnancy". In: *Complementary Therapies in Medicine* 23(04): 509–515. Doi: 10.1016/j.ctim.2015.05.002

Chen PJ, Yang L, Chou CC, Li CC, Chang YC, Liaw JJ (2017) "Effects of prenatal yoga on women's stress and immune function across pregnancy: A randomized controlled trial". In: *Complementary Therapies in Medicine*, April 2017, 31: 109–117. https://doi.org/10.1016/j.ctim.2017.03.003

Dennis CL Ross LE, Grigoriadis S (2007) Psychosocial and psychological interventions for treating antenatal depression. https://doi.org/10.1002/14651858.CD006309.pub2

Dietz P, Watson ED, Sattler MC, Ruf W, Titze S, van Poppel M (2016) "The influence of physical activity during pregnancy on maternal, fetal or infant heart rate variability: a systematic review". In: *BMC Pregnancy and Childbirth* 16: 326. doi: 10.1186/s12884-016-1121-7

Dilcher B (2021) "Erik: Case study of an experienced one twin loss". In: Evertz K, Janus L, Linder R (eds.) *Handbook of prenatal and perinatal psychology - Integrating research and practice*. Springer Nature, Heidelberg, New York, 333–336.

Emerson W (2021) *Birth trauma. The effects of modern obstetrics on the human psyche*. Mattes, Heidelberg.

Evertz K (2016) "A visual exploration of psychodynamics in problematic pregnancies: Case studies in analytic-aesthetic art therapy". In: *Journal of Prenatal and Perinatal Psychology and Health* Winter 2016; 31(2): 107–133.

Evertz K (2020a) "The inner child or the "inner child"? - Transgenerational and prenatal trauma layers". In: *Forum für Kunsttherapien, Zeitschrift des Fachverbandes für Gestaltende Psychotherapie und Kunsttherapie GPK*, Aarburg, Switzerland, 30–36.

Evertz K (2020b) "The inner child or the "inner child"? Confusion during pregnancy and its lifelong consequences". In: Gouni O et al. (eds.) *Change - Birthing & parenting at times of crisis*. Cosmoanelixis, Athens, 2021, 293–334.

Evertz K (2021) "A visual exploration of psychodynamics in problematic pregnancies: Case studies in analytic-aesthetic art therapy". In: Evertz K et al. (eds.) *Handbook for prenatal psychology - Integrating research and practice*. Springer, Heidelberg, New York, 309–331.

Evertz K (2022) "Die Welt neu spüren - Die transgenerational-systemisch und pränatal fundierte methodenintegrative Psychotherapie - Integrative Kunst- und Körpertherapie". In: Klippel-Heidekrüger M, Janus L (eds.) *Vielfältige Zugänge zum vorsprachlichen und geburtlichen Erleben*. Mattes Verlag, Heidelberg, 271–292.

Evertz K, Janus L, Linder R (2021) *Handbook of prenatal and perinatal psychology - Integrating research and practice*. Springer Nature, Heidelberg, New York.

Field T, Hemandez-Reif M, Hart S, Theakston H, Schanberg S, Kuhn C (1999) "Pregnant women benefit from massage therapy". In: *Journal of Psychosomatic Obstetrics & Gynecology* 20(1): 31–38. https://doi.org/10.3109/01674829909075574

Frederiksen Y, Farver-Vestergaard I, Skovgård NG (2015) "Efficacy of psychosocial interventions for psychological and pregnancy outcomes in infertile women and men: a systematic review and meta-analysis". In: *BMJ Open* 5: e006592. doi: 10.1136/bmjopen-2014-006592

Fredrickson BL, Boulton AJ, Firestine AM (2017) Positive emotion correlates of meditation practice: a comparison of mindfulness meditation and loving-kindness meditation. In: *Mindfulness* 8: 1623–1633. https://doi.org/10.1007/s12671-017-0735-9

Gluckman P, Hanson M, Seng CY, Bardsley A. (2015) *Nutrition and Lifestyle for Pregnancy and Breastfeeding*. Oxford University Press, Oxford.

Goertz-Schroth A, Schroth G, Phillips R (2023) "Prenatal bonding (BA) as a breakthrough in improving pregnancy, birth, and postpartum outcomes". In: *Journal for Prenatal and Perinatal Psychology and Health*, Spring 202337(1): 1–21.

Grote N, Bledsoe SE (2006) "Treating depression during pregnancy and the postpartum: A preliminary meta-analysis". In: *Research on Social Work Practice* 16(2): 109–120. https://doi.org/10.1177/1049731505282202

Grote N, Katon WJ, Russo JE, Lohr MJ, Curran M, Galvin E, Carson K (2015) "Collaborative care for perinatal depression in socio-economically disadvantaged women: A randomised trial". In: *Depress Anxiety* 2015 November; 32(11): 821–834. Published online 2015 September 8. https://doi.org/10.1002/da.22405

Hüning B, Jäkel J (2021) Prematurity and long-term consequences up to school age. https://doi.org/10.1026/0942-5403/A000326

Legrand F, Grévin-Laroche C, Josse E, Polidori G, Quinart H, Taïar R (2017) "Effects of hypnosis during pregnancy: A psychophysiological study on maternal stress". In: *Medical Hypotheses* May 2017, 102: 123–127. https://doi.org/10.1016/j.mehy.2017.03.026

Linder R (2021a) "Early care networks in Germany and initiation of the Pforzheim study". In: Evertz K, Janus L, Linder R (eds.) *Handbook of prenatal and perinatal psychology - Integrating research and practice*. Springer Nature, Heidelberg, New York, 627–672.

Linder R (2021b) "On the psychodynamics of Preeclampsia and HELLP Syndrome". In: Evertz K, Janus L, Linder R (eds.) *Handbook of prenatal and perinatal psychology - Integrating research and practice*. Springer Nature, Heidelberg, New York, 291–308.

Linder R (2024) Personal communication. Unpublished

Linderkamp O (2021a) "Dealing with the healthy and premature child in times of Corona". In: Reiß R et al. (eds.) *Kindheit ist politisch - die Bedeutung der frühen Kindheit für die Konflikt- und Handlungsfähigkeit in der Gesellschaft. Jahrbuch für psychohistorische Forschung,* vol. 21. Mattes, Heidelberg, 135–157.

Linderkamp O (2021b) "Family-centered individualised developmental care of the preterm baby". In: Evertz K, Janus L, Linder R (eds.) *Handbook of prenatal and perinatal psychology - Integrating research and practice*. Springer Nature, Heidelberg, New York, 377–390.

Marc I, Toureche N, Ernst E, Hodnett ED, Blanchet C, Dodin S, Njoya MM. (2011) "Mind-body interventions during pregnancy for preventing or treating women's anxiety". In: *Cochrane Database of Systematic Reviews* 2011(7): CD007559. https://doi:10.1002/14651858.CD007559.pub2.

Matvienko-Sikar K, Dockray S (2017) "Effects of a novel positive psychological intervention on prenatal stress and well-being: A pilot randomised controlled trial". In: *Women and Birth* 30(2): e111–e118. https://doi.org/10.1016/j.wombi.2016.10.003

Narendran S, Nagarathna R, Narendran V, Gunasheela S, Nagendra HRR (2005) "Efficacy of yoga on pregnancy outcome". In: *Journal of Alternative and Complementary Medicine* 11(2): 237–244. https://doi: 10.1089/acm.2005.11.237.

Ott M, Singer M, Bliem HR, Schubert C (2021) "Prenatal psychoneuroimmunology". In: Evertz K, Janus L, Linder R (eds.) *Handbook of prenatal and perinatal psychology*. Springer, New York, S. 115–158.

Pan WL, Gau ML, Lee TY, Jou HJ, Liu CY, Wen TK (2019) "Mindfulness-based programme on the psychological health of pregnant women". In: *Women and Birth* February 2019, 32(1): e102–e109. https://doi.org/10.1016/j.wombi.2018.04.018

Pro Familia (2024) https://www.profamilia.de/angebote-vor-ort/nordrhein-westfalen/koeln-zentrum/depressionen-waehrend-und-nach-der-schwangerschaft

Rath W, Baltzer J (2005) *Diseases during pregnancy*. Stuttgart, Thieme

Schroth G (2021) "Postpartum mood disorders: Prevention by prenatal bonding (BA)". In: Evertz, K, Janus L, Linder R (eds.) *Handbook of prenatal and perinatal psychology*. Springer Nature, Switzerland, 611–618.

Shimada BMO, da Silva Oliveira Menezes dos Santos M, Cabral MA, Silva VO, Vagetti GC (2020) "Interventions among Pregnant Women in the Field of Music Therapy: A Systematic Review". In: *Revista Brasileira de Ginecologia e Obstetrícia* 2021; 43(5):403–413. https://doi.org/10.1055/s-0041-1731924.

Steller J, Goerke K (2018) "Pregnancy". In: Goerke Kay, Steller Joachim, Valet Axel (eds.) *Clinic guide gynaecology obstetrics* (Tenth Edition), Clinic Guide. Munich, Urban & Fischer, 107–183.

Tomfor-Madsen LM, Campbell TS, Giesbrecht GF, Letourneau NL, Carlson LE, Madsen JW, Dimidjian S (2016) "Mindfulness-based cognitive therapy for psychological distress in pregnancy: study protocol for a randomized controlled trial". In: *Trials* 17: 498. Doi: 10.1186/s13063-016-1601-0

Urizar GG (2023) "Chapter 6 - Stress and cortisol regulation during pregnancy: Implications for cognitive behavioral stress management among low-income women". In: *Handbook of Lifespan Cognitive Behavioral Therapy - Childhood, Adolescence, Pregnancy, Adulthood, and Aging*, 65–77. https://doi.org/10.1016/B978-0-323-85757-4.00034-1

van Willenswaard KC, Lynn F, McNeill J, et al. (2017) "Music interventions to reduce stress and anxiety in pregnancy: a systematic review and meta-analysis". In: *BMC Psychiatry* 17(01): 271. Doi: 10.1186/s12888-017-1432-x

Verny T (2003) *The baby of tomorrow*. Zweitausendeins, Frankfurt.

Vieten C, Astin J (2008) "Effects of a mindfulness-based intervention during pregnancy on prenatal stress and mood: Results of a pilot study". In: *Archives of Women's Mental Health* 11(1): 67–74. https://doi.org/10.1007/s00737-008-0214-3

Weintraub P (1992) *Life before birth. A nine-month programme for you and your unborn child*. Two thousand and one, Frankfurt.

Wessel J, Endrikat J, Buscher U (2002) "Frequency of denial of pregnancy; results and epidemiological significance of a 1-year prospective study in Berlin". In: *Acta Obstetrica et Gynecologica Scandinavica* 81: 1021–1027.

WHO recommendations for care of the preterm or low-birth-weight infant (2022). https://www.who.int/publications/i/item/9

Wikipedia (2024) https://de.wikipedia.org/wiki/Totgeburt

Woods SM Melville JL, Guo Y, Fan MY, Gavin A (2010) "Psychosocial stress during pregnancy". In: *American Journal of Obstetrics Gynecology* January; 202(1): 61–67. https://doi:10.1016/j.ajog.2009.07.041. Epub 2009 September 20.

9

PRENATAL PSYCHOTHERAPY

Prenatal psychotraumatology

Psychotherapy today

Modern psychotherapy can look back on over 120 years of history and has scientifically researched that all mental disorders and illnesses are essentially based on an interplay between genetic-epigenetic predispositions and prenatal/early postnatal negative experiences and influences. The evidence is repeatedly provided in line with and based on the results of prenatal extended developmental psychology and prenatal-based attachment research. In therapeutic work, transgenerational, periconceptional, prenatal, perinatal and postnatal traumatic stress can be differentiated for the first time. Prenatal psychotraumatology is therefore the interface for the diagnosis of mental disorders in their aetiology between hereditary and personal biographical experiences. The differentiated clarification of the trauma stratification of a biography is essential for sustainable healing processes (Hochauf 2007, 2021; Evertz 2020, 2021, 2022; Janus 2013).

Lambert and Barley summarise the basic findings of general psychotherapy research on the therapeutic relationship and therapy effects:

- Psychotherapy in general is effective. The average treated patient feels better than 80% of untreated people
    - 15% expectation effects (placebo)
    - 15% Method
    - 30% Therapeutic relationship
    - 40% Extratherapeutic changes

(Lambert & Barley 2001)

DOI: 10.4324/9781003480242-9

Psychotherapy initially means creating an emotionally safe space for issues that represent a crisis in the patient's life. How do patients answer the question about the conditions of a good therapeutic relationship?

1	Trust	59%
2	Empathy	51%
3	Sympathy	33%
4	Always available/enough time	32%
5	Showing possible solutions to problems	29%
6	Respect	29%
7	Being a good listener	25%
8	Openness	20%

From the patient's perspective, 100 inpatients with neurotic disorders (Hermer & Röhrle 2008, p. 72).

The patient expects help and support in their everyday problems (behavioural therapy) and also in their deeper life conflicts and mental illnesses (depth psychology). The psychotherapeutic setting must be adapted depending on the extent of the psychological stress and disorder. However, the constitutional emotional possibilities are also always addressed. As a rule, the current crisis also intensifies the conflict-laden and unresolved life issues. A strong indicator of a good prognosis is emotional stability and resource abilities or, in other words, the continuum of basic trust.

Treasures of early good bonding are:

– Ability to love
– Bonding and relationship skills
– Self-efficacy
– Good body awareness
– Safe body image and body schema
– Capacity for ambivalence – mentalisation
– Dealing with cognitive dissonance
– Value relativism
– Paradox tolerance
– Uncertainty tolerance
– Humour
– Learning to accept life as a creation of meaning – the meaning of life is life itself and its creation

In every psychotherapy session, the aim is to build on the patient's resources and, after initial phases of stabilisation, to alternate between the phases of discovery work. From a neurobiological point of view, the main effective factor is the therapeutic relationship: the therapeutic alliance. It can cause massive releases of oxytocin and endogenous opioids, which trigger a noticeable improvement in symptoms. In mild cases of mental disorder, this can lead to good treatment success.

> In more severe mental disorders, which are based on an interaction between genetic-epigenetic predispositions, prenatal and early childhood negative experiences, a second and more "implicit" phase of therapy is necessary, in which structural changes must occur in the basal ganglia. New neurones are formed not only in the hippocampus, but also in the striatum, more precisely in the caudate nucleus and the putamen. This adult neurogenesis is disrupted by stress and promoted by oxytocin. The therapeutic alliance is the non-specific helper here.
>
> *(Roth 2014, p. 380)*

In prenatal psychotherapy, the therapeutic alliance becomes a specific helper through the conscious integration of the prenatal bonding levels. The therapeutic relationship as the main effective factor in the relationship is perceived by both sides as the warmth of a human relationship. For the patient, it is often a question of relearning what a human relationship can actually be. The disappointments and suffering of people traumatised in childhood indicate the lack of security and protection, empathy and warmth in their previous lives. Also the inability to enter into loving relationships, even though they are desired. Transference and counter-transference are important instruments for recognising the longing, pain, anger and grief of the inner child and exploring the possibilities of growing up again.

Prenatal psychotherapy – prenatal psychotraumatology

Basically, it can be said that sound psychotherapeutic training is a prerequisite for expanding this to include the pre- and perinatal dimension, as there are still few training and further education opportunities for complete prenatal psychotherapy (Evertz 2022).

A fundamental extension of previous psychotherapy is both the expansion of therapeutic knowledge and the expansion of therapeutic means. Body-psychotherapeutic methods, psychodramatic and music-therapeutic methods, art-psychotherapeutic methods and depth-psychology-based forms of psychotherapy can all complement each other to form a prenatal-based psychotherapy.

In therapeutic groups, the more and deeper each participant opens up and reveals something of her own story and emotional life, the more tangible and palpable the community experience becomes. In contrast to human groups, which discuss factual issues and supposedly only deal with them on an intellectual level, therapeutic groups are concerned with the issues of coping with life in times of crisis and illness, including the subjective sensitivities, feelings, behaviour and thinking of the participants. These groups are generally based on trust, as the work is subject to stricter protective regulations, such as confidentiality, and a therapeutic objective.

In therapeutic groups, a group dynamic develops, a motherly-fatherly field (Fink), in which increased empathy is possible. The deeper the topics touch on the basic conditions of human existence and the more they actually become possible in the emotional opening, the deeper the relationship between the participants becomes. Suddenly it is about everyone bearing witness to the conditions of their own existence and the conditions for human coexistence in general. This is only possible if the setting is clearly appreciative, caring, protective, equalising and authentic.

This becomes even stronger the more the exchange takes place not only in verbal form but also non-verbally, e.g. via painted pictures, bodywork, scenic representations (family constellations, confronting issues, etc.), music and dance (music and dance therapy) and playful forms of expression (psychodrama, theatre therapy), etc. The more seriously a therapist and/or therapeutic group endeavours to perceive and understand the other person's life story, the more the person's longing for closeness and being seen, for being taken seriously and understood, for healing and security can be fulfilled, at least to some extent.

And the smaller the participant's inner wounded child is, the more it is truly recognised and acknowledged: from the very first cell.

Where can you talk about the fact that there is a deep biographical pain about the fact that the parents did not actually want a child at that time, that they wanted a different sex for the child, that there were abortion attempts or abortion fantasies? That the parents were unhappy with each other. That there were losses, separations, violence, accidents, fear and panic, depression and other hardships for the mother or father during the pregnancy.

The statement by many participants alone that they are disclosing these facts to a group for the first time, that no one else knows, that they have tried to suppress it for a long time, or that they often only realise during the work that there is an early trauma, makes it clear that the deeper the life issues are, the more profound the communion made possible by the setting.

Case vignette: transgenerationality

Case vignette: A 60-year-old woman, who had been confronted with cancer for more than 20 years of her life, fell into a deep emotional layer of great physical and emotional coldness during a body therapy regression. Where she had just felt safe and relaxed in a lying position, she suddenly said: "I'm sinking deeper and deeper and I'm getting scared, it's getting so cold……" Even adding blankets did not change the feeling of cold. When asked if there were any images to go with this terrifying feeling of cold, she said it had something to do with her father and Russia. Her father was a soldier in the German "Barbarossa" campaign against the Soviet Union. But it would be something else than the horrors of war and the cold traumas in the Russian winter that her father had suffered……. and then she was able to report that her father, as a survivor of the Russian campaign, learnt on the way home after many hardships that his pregnant wife and their three-year-old daughter had been killed in a bombing raid on a train……… and never spoke about it later. Her father had then remarried and had her and her brother as "new" children. But he was never really available for her and her brother. There was always a layer of coldness. She always felt that her cancer was a layer of coldness: that she couldn't feel what was happening to her and that the cancer was an expression of the inner stress of "not feeling". With strong emotional sensations, she regained more warmth for herself in the further bodywork and the feeling that she had always carried her father's enormous pain associated with cold and death within her and could now finally leave it behind, as if in the depths of a grave in winter. She now felt that this pain was not really hers, but that she had always thought it was hers….. "from the beginning". Now she could rise up and felt very light and liberated (Such settings last between 45 minutes and three hours and only a brief insight into the differentiated emotional work can be given here).

In the "father journeys", i.e. guided body-psychotherapeutic regressions into the conception, we very often experience how the traumas from the father's life story can be felt like the first introjects, whereas in the previous life they had always been perceived as something separate. This emotional differentiation allows an inner regulation of large emotional mixtures that previously seemed indissoluble. The same happens in the "mother journeys" in relation to the mother's life story. An affective clarification and purification take place, so to speak. The agonising aspect of transgenerational traumatic information in the psyche is its depressive indissolubility, which can only be ended when it is possible to sort out emotionally what it is all about. The decisive difference in psychotherapy is whether we have experienced a trauma in our own biography or whether we consider a transgenerational trauma to be our own experience. Healing therefore takes place in the physical and emotional perception of where a pain, a disorder or a conflict actually originated. Only then can an integrative understanding be achieved cognitively: a trauma from one's own history can be processed and often healed, a trauma from the parents' generation can only be "returned".

Detachment from the maternal and/or paternal introject, i.e. from an unresolved psychological part inherited from the mother/father, is therapeutically an important level of healing of transgenerational and prenatal relationship conflicts that determine all later relationships in life.

A 50-year-old woman is working on her relationship and commitment anxiety. She suffers from physical and psychological symptoms such as panic attacks and high blood pressure. After lengthy depth psychology work she comes to the realisation that she has already suffered intrauterine from not being seen by her mother.

For the first time, in a bodywork session with two other women, she can allow touch on her back and feet and allow herself to be involved and then allow the feeling that for the first time she can feel the ambivalent mother introject in simultaneity: on the one hand, everything is good and she feels completely close and safe and at the same time she is completely alone: in other words, an actually crazy feeling of simultaneous closeness and relationship and loneliness. The resolution lies in the fact that the mother was pregnant with her and was also able to be affectionate but also partially fell out of contact with the child and fell into her depression, into her unresolved grief for a stillborn child before the current pregnancy. The client's inner child always felt this as abandonment and not knowing whether the mother would come back into contact or whether she would have to stay behind in darkness and loneliness. She tried to save and hold on to the feeling of closeness, not being allowed to move so as not to tip back into the fear-inducing abandonment (Figures 9.1–9.3).

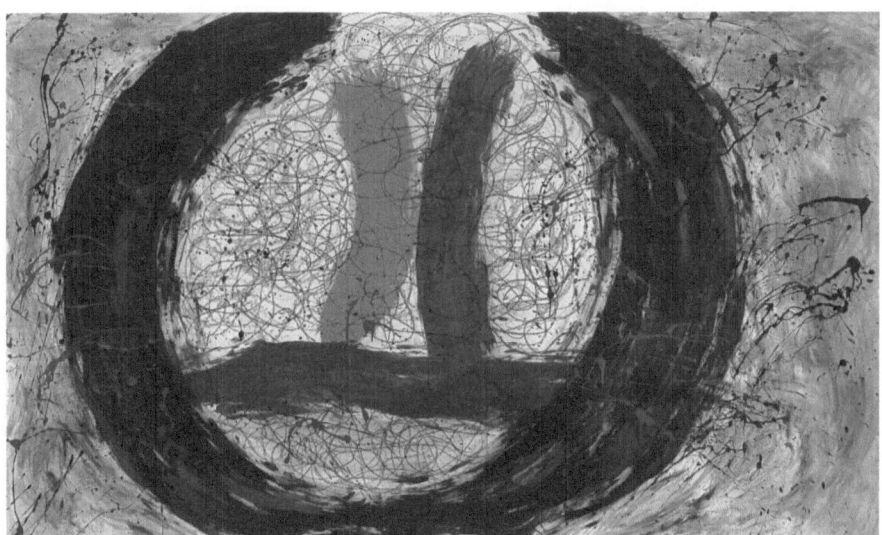

FIGURE 9.1   She can express the feelings of this fundamental maternal conflict in a large picture.

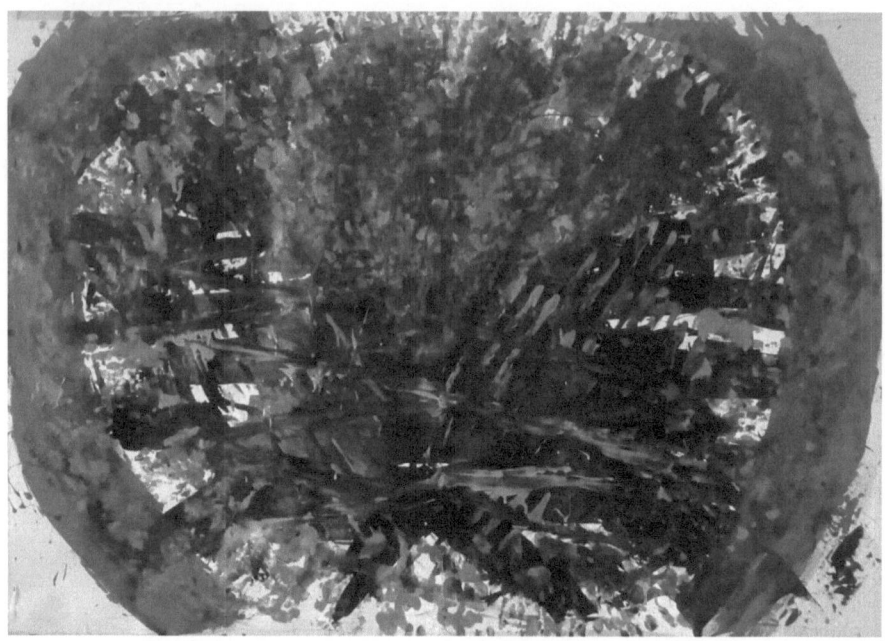

FIGURE 9.2 In another picture a few weeks later, she can paint this picture after falling in love with a man again. A fully perfused placenta as a positive sign of the possibility of a strong relationship, despite and with the conflict-laden levels.

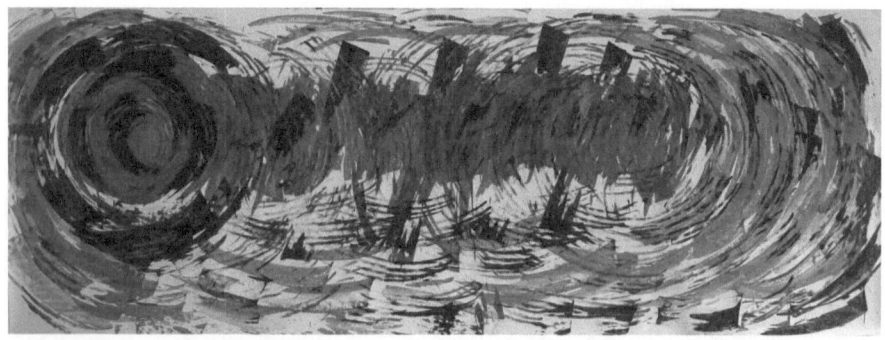

FIGURE 9.3 In a third large picture (approx. 5 × 2 m), again a few weeks later after a regressive birth experience, there is a great integrative power to be able to integrate the masculine and the feminine.

Overcoming early traumas of loss is achieved in therapy by re-experiencing the pain but here in a protected space with the parallelisation of the therapeutic timelines so that the old pain does not have to be repeated in the future. It can finally be categorised where it actually happened and only then can it be left behind. If this clarification does not take place, many people repeat the early pain of loss again and again, for example, by falling in love with the very people they do not actually want, i.e. by whom they are not actually wanted. So where only the rejecting or pain-filled part of the early mother makes up the attraction, instead of the affirming and joyful part of the mother.

It is not about a pregnant woman not being in conscious contact with her child at times, but about a serious lack of contact due to a personality disorder, anxiety disorder or depression in the mother, which can have an overwhelmingly anxiety-inducing effect on the child. The child can distinguish very well between a normal everyday stress of the mother, in which she goes to work and at times does not think about her pregnancy and does not feel close to her child, and a real traumatic loss of contact due to a childhood trauma of the mother or a current mental or physical illness or other significant distress of the mother.

The bio-psycho-social model of prenatal psychology and the model of ontological consciousness imply that the early imprints are the strongest, simply because the basic structures of the entire organism (organs, CNS, immune system, hormonal system, etc.) are formed here and are more difficult to reshape than later levels of growth.

The cell and body memory of every human being "knows" everything that has ever affected the body and can remember it in many different ways but not necessarily consciously. There is no person who is not in constant interaction with other people from the very beginning.

However, a person's first relationship is with their parents. The compatibility and incompatibility of parents are the most important basic characteristics for bio-psycho-social development and the individual's own new learning of relationships and attachment.

Therapy methods

For many decades, therapy methods have been tried and tested with which patients could be led into a deep regression back to the beginning of their lives in a protected setting. All responsible therapists realise that it is easy to lead people into a regression, but that it is crucial to be able to accompany people in the regression competently and with therapeutic empathy and an overview of trauma so that corrective experiences can take place. The patient must become aware of the original context of a primary memory in order to be able to integrate the separated memory system, that which has been split off. With LSD and hypnosis, for example, this is only possible to a limited extent because the patient's consciousness does not clearly experience the regression taking place here. Breathing techniques and other body-psychotherapeutic options are more conscious and effective.

Frank Lake began using LSD 25 in psychotherapy in 1954, Stanislav Grof in 1956 (Lake 1981; Grof 1990). Lake gave it up in 1969. His view was also shared by Janov: "What LSD does not do is facilitate connections that are solid. And only connections bring about lasting change." (Janov 1973) He also avoided the use of LSD, as did Konrad Stettbacher (1991), the primary therapist of the author Alice Miller (1991) in Switzerland. Influenced by Reich's technique and bioenergetics, Lake found that a "pattern of deep breathing that we came across" surpassed the effects of LSD. Patients were better able to recognise their powerful physical experience as a reliving of their birth or their devastating sense of rejection in the womb. Lake instructed, "Breathe up into your strength, down into your weakness," pausing slightly each time the lungs were full or empty. This breathing brought the brain into the theta rhythm. The theta rhythm is more pronounced in very young children than in adults. It seems to establish a link between conscious and subconscious thought (Lake 1981; Pelletier 1978). The theta rhythm is associated with sleepiness and hypnagogic imagination, while the alpha rhythm is associated with meditation and mysticism (Johnston 1974). Lake said (Lake 1981):

(This breathing method) promotes a faithful grasp and "contextualisation" of the intrauterine experience. Under LSD, the subject avoids the actual horrors or joys of the foetus itself and evades the realisation that this is happening to them in the context of their own mother's womb.... The actual experience of the individual has been relegated to the realm of myth and dream-like sequences that occur in symbolically represented religious conflicts and liberations. The work of Stanislav Grof, who continues to use LSD, confirms this observation.

What about the transmission? Lake explained (Lake 1981):

We are looking for a 'therapeutic alliance' with an adult, not a parent-child transfer.... We facilitate his direct access to his own feelings, to a time when he was in direct contact with the mother's personality, and through her with the father's and their otherworldly world.

(House 1999, p. 444)

Ultimately, the problem of transference of early references was only solved by Renate Hochauf with her technique of parallelisation, while in many therapies early transference is classified as persistent resistance or disturbance of the patient. This is a background for the inconclusiveness of pre-linguistic transference because it cannot be recognised and also cannot be processed without the prenatal psychological level (Hochauf 2007, 2021).

The structure of severe personality disorders is primarily characterised by a high proportion of pre-symbolic representations and dissociative defence patterns. The background to this is usually early traumatic experiences that result in structural deficits. They originate from the time before, during and after birth. Central symbolisation processes may then have been blocked and hindered early on in the course of structure formation.

(Hochauf 2023)

As soon as a therapeutic field is opened up that allows for the transgenerational, prenatal and perinatal psychic fields, intensive work on the inner and outer understanding of major life contexts arises in individual psychotherapeutic work or in group therapeutic work with people.

In a large drawing, a 70-year-old therapist and training participant expresses the question of how the loneliness she feels now and has felt for most of her life is connected to her earliest impressions. An early cell shape lies on a field of black arrows and attacks and ends in a phalanx of five vertical red arrows pointing to a smaller blue circular shape. It poses the question of how a delicate, warm and large form became a small contracted blue form through unfavourable influences (Figures 9.4 and 9.5).

She gives an answer in the second picture. She writes:

In the body therapy self-awareness session, the image of Moses in the wicker basket, a foundling described in the Bible, appeared to me. This represents the feeling of being lost as a fundamental attitude to life for both me and my father.

My father was born out of wedlock. His mother died shortly after giving birth. His father gave the baby to a foster family, where he was inadequately cared for. He never knew where he belonged.

The author of the picture has inherited her father's terrible experience of loneliness, not only losing her mother at such an early age but also being placed in a strange and rejecting family, and can now take her own inner child in her arms, detached from the father's abandonment. In this second picture, she thus detaches herself from the father's introject!

All people who confront their origins and origins in therapeutic groups come to the conclusion that many things in their feelings and thoughts now come together and connect all at once, as if they were learning to understand their lives anew. This is felt very strongly emotionally, many tears flow, a lot of closeness and support and protection is needed, but it has a very healing and lasting effect on the current life situation and current crises and stagnation. Identity is strengthened when one's own life story is understood more comprehensively and can be felt.

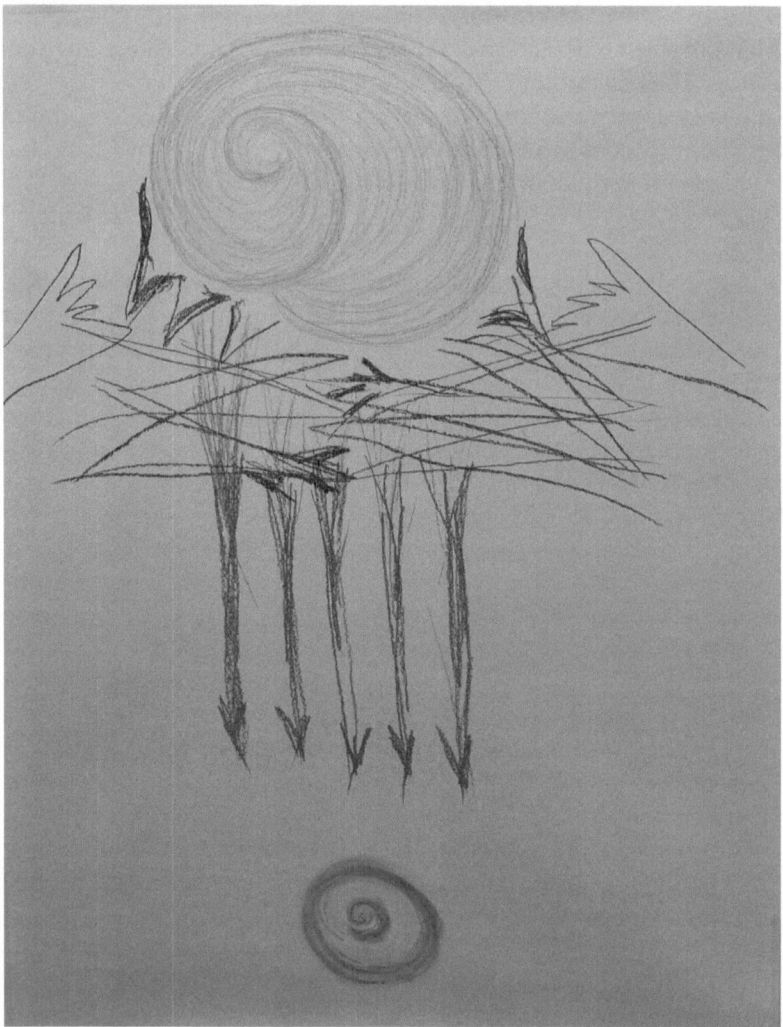

FIGURE 9.4

This bio-psycho-social field, I also call it ontological awareness, of a person's entire existence from conception to the present, can be utilised therapeutically today. It is not only a question of long-term, deep-psychological forms of therapy in which these themes are slowly and carefully developed, but this knowledge can also be utilised in low-threshold therapeutic levels. The top priority is, of course, the safety of the therapeutic setting in order to prevent re-traumatisation. In pregnancy counselling and maternity care, this knowledge can be used even with one-off psychotherapeutic interventions in gynaecological-psychotherapeutic practice to safeguard endangered

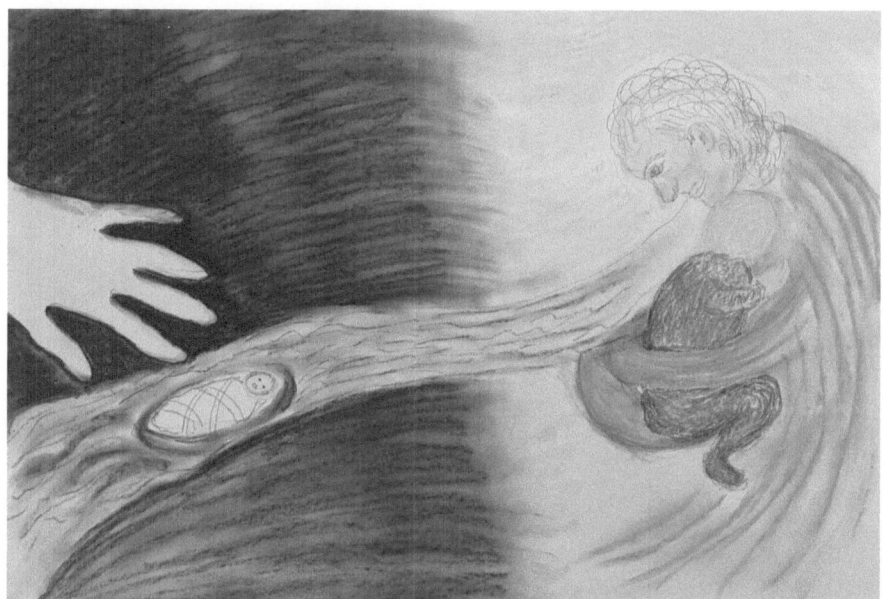

FIGURE 9.5

pregnancies, in which the pregnant woman can reflect on her own pregnancy and birth and also that of the mother and can free herself from old traumatisation and repetition constraints of the female line of the family system (Figure 9.6) (Linder 2021).

Prenatal traumatisation refers to traumatic experiences that occur during pregnancy and can affect the unborn child. Here is a list of possibilities of prenatal traumatisation:

1 Maternal stress: If the pregnant mother is exposed to high levels of stress, this can have an impact on the unborn child. Chronic stress can lead to increased cortisol levels, which can increase the risk of developmental problems.
2 Violence or abuse: If the pregnant mother experiences violence or abuse, this can lead to traumatic experiences for the unborn child. The effects can be of an emotional or physical nature.
3 Substance use: The consumption of alcohol, drugs or nicotine during pregnancy can lead to prenatal traumatisation and increase the risk of developmental disorders.
4 Medical interventions: In some cases, medical interventions during pregnancy can be traumatic, such as invasive examinations or complications during labour.

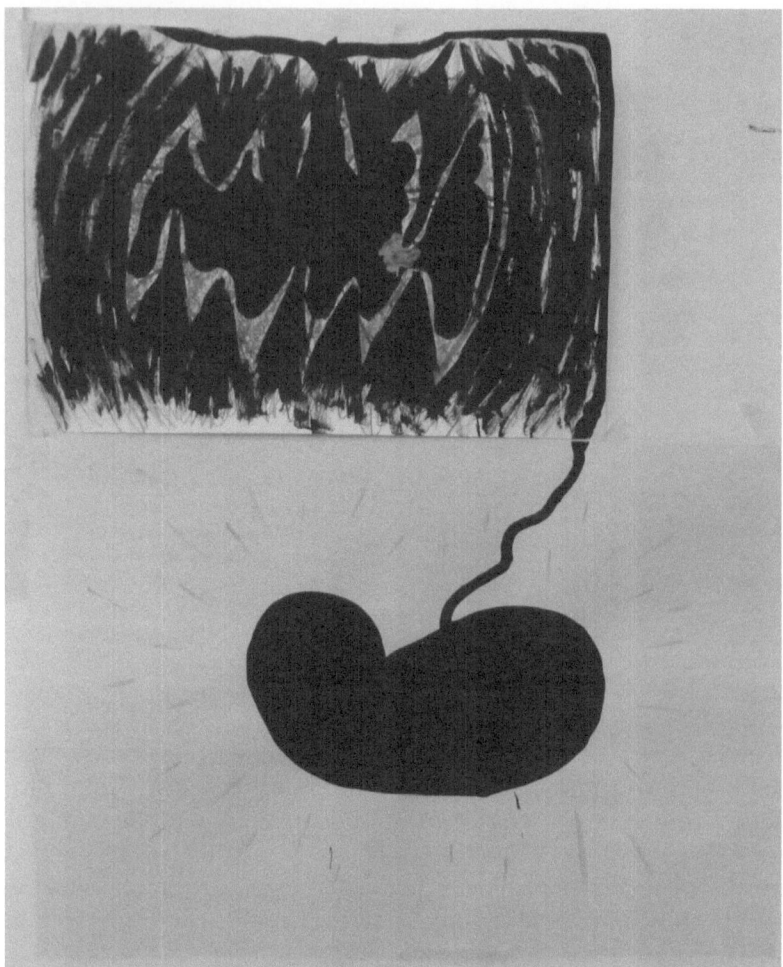

FIGURE 9.6   "Fighting or threatening placenta" – the placental receptivity of many of the mother's hormonal messages is well documented biologically and psychologically (Ott et al. 2021) (Painting of a 45-year-old woman).

5 Loss or separation: If the pregnant mother experiences a loss or is separated from an important attachment figure, this can lead to prenatal traumatisation.
6 Unhealthy environment: An unfavourable environment during pregnancy, such as poverty, lack of nutrition or poor living conditions, can increase the risk of prenatal traumatisation.
7 Illness or infections: Pregnant women suffering from serious illnesses or infections can cause traumatic experiences for the unborn child.

8 Accident or injury: If the pregnant mother has an accident or injures herself, this can lead to prenatal traumatisation.
9 Unintended pregnancy: An unwanted pregnancy can lead to emotional stress that can affect the unborn child.
10 Mental illness of the mother: If the pregnant mother suffers from a mental illness, this can lead to prenatal traumatisation, as emotional stability may be impaired.
11 Significant psychosocial stress of the father or in the entire family system naturally always has the same effect on the pregnant mother and the child.

It is always important to note that prenatal traumatisation can vary greatly from person to person and is not always obvious.

The treatment of prenatal traumatisation involves a deep empathic layer of perception on the part of the therapist, who has learned to empathise with early childhood and prenatal layers of experience through his own training and self-awareness.

In prenatal psychotherapy, a distinction must therefore be made as to when we speak of "introjects", defined as life-restricting, development-inhibiting, disease-causing or disease-promoting, etc., biological-psychological patterns from the unresolved traumas of the parents that can impair ontogenesis from the beginning of pregnancy and peri- and postnatally. We need to differentiate between biological-psychological patterns from the unresolved traumas of the parents, which can affect ontogenesis from the beginning of pregnancy and peri- and postnatally, and when we speak of the influencing factors of the "genetic inheritance" as a risk potential that becomes effective during conception in the unique mixture of maternal and paternal DNA. From conception onwards, this risk potential can be influenced and modified in a variety of ways by the epigenetic factors that emerge – both to reinforce and to mitigate transgenerational crisis information.

As subjective qualities of experience, we can now learn to distinguish between these two levels in deep regressive settings (Evertz et al. 2021; Evertz 2022; Terry 2014; Emerson 2021): genetic inheritance and our own ontogenesis from the very first cell. The very first cellular memory systems of humans in their first weeks of life grow seamlessly and generatively into the first neuronal memory systems (Linderkamp 2014; Verdult 2014). From this perspective, no information from life experience is ever lost in living systems. And from a philosophical perspective, it is clear that, ontologically speaking, there is no separation between the biological and the psychological anyway.

An example from everyday practice: If the father and mother both experienced a trauma in their childhood, e.g. the father the loss of two younger siblings (drowned while ice skating) and the mother the loss of her own mother, and both parents have not been able to process this traumatic shock of their childhood in their lives or have hardly been able to do so, then it can be assumed that the child will firstly the unresolved traumas of the parents are passed on as a cell-chemical message in the DNA of the parents and, secondly, that the child senses this unresolved (inaccessible, solidified, fear-inducing, dead, depressive) in the maternal space in the bond to the mother (and to the father, mediated via the mother) from the very beginning and initially considers it to be its own! And must take it for its own, because there is no clarifying authority in the parents. The introject would therefore be an unresolved death threat.

As a rule, this introject is of course permanently "fed" by the parents' interaction with the postnatal child. The baby and toddler will also always sense this inaccessible or fear-inducing layer in the parents and orientate their own lives accordingly: e.g. in the form of an expectation of catastrophe and paranoia (so-called cry babies usually unconsciously express the parents' "inability to cry" about their own repressed pain).

Prenatal-based psychotherapeutic work in adult and paediatric therapy now aims to clear up these old and perceived "confusions" in order to heal existing mental disorders and illnesses or psychological suffering as far as possible.

Janus formulates general conclusions from this for psychotherapy and psychosomatics:

- Detailed anamnestic clarification of prenatal and obstetric conditions.
- Expansion of diagnostic-therapeutic perception for the descendants of pre-linguistic experience.
- Consideration of the descendants of prenatal and birth bonding dynamics in the therapeutic process.
- Observing the primary conditions for realistic goal setting and planning (Janus 2013).
- Clarification of trauma stratification, differentiation of transgenerational, periconceptional, prenatal, perinatal and early postnatal traumatisation or severe psychosocial stress (Evertz 2020, 2022; Hochauf 2007, 2021).

The confusion between self-experience and transgenerational life experiences may be lifelong psychodynamic work: on the one hand, there is the "drive-dynamic" demand to realise one's own potential (Balint); on the other hand, there are the "restraining forces" (introjects) of "love for the trauma-tised "inner children" in the parents", i.e. not wanting (being able) to leave them alone in their childhood destinies. As these connections usually remain unconscious, it becomes clear how many atmospheric disturbances there are in family relationships for which there is no actual blame, but for which there is often only a struggle over levels of guilt....... and, in the worst case, new traumatisation is generated (Hirsch 2004).

When the child becomes an adult, it remains in a certain sense below its potential in life if it has to expend a great deal of emotional energy on the parentified parts. Of course, this task of providing lifelong (psychological) care for the parents can also lead to the development of special talents, such as those increasingly found in the so-called helping professions in medicine, therapy, social work, education, etc. However, the system often breaks down prematurely, as the task will always be too much for the child as well as for the adult child: a child can never heal the traumas of the parents, they can only do this themselves (Figure 9.7).

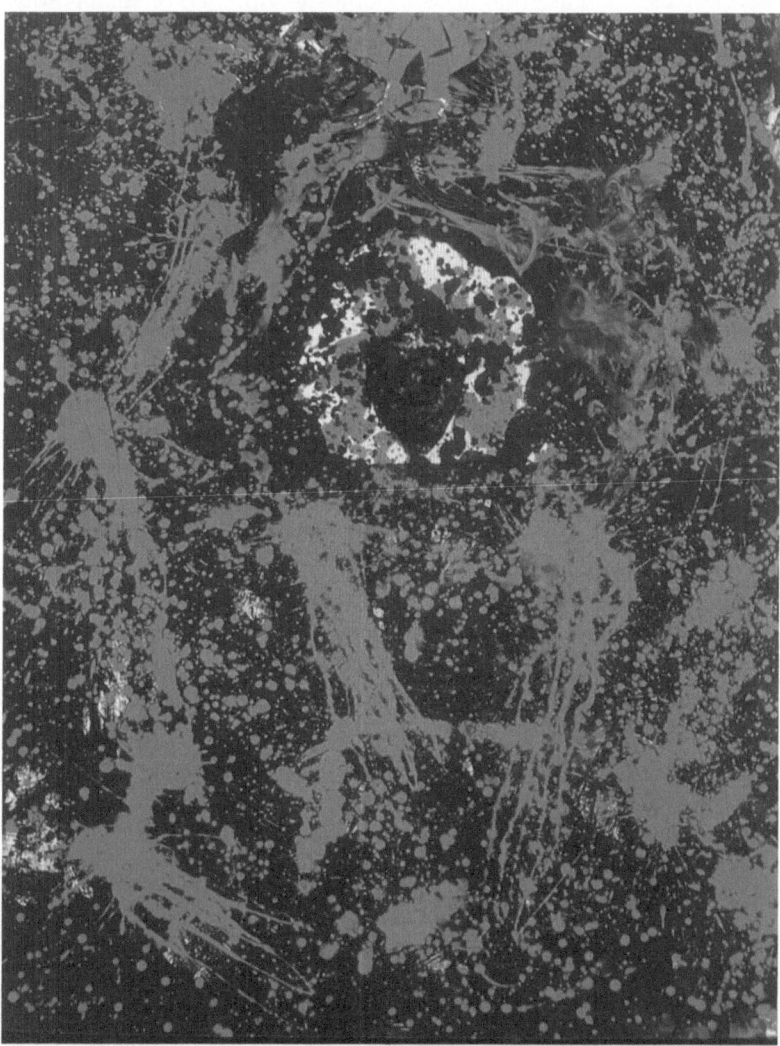

FIGURE 9.7 "Prenatal stress", painting by a 60-year-old artist.

Aspects of trauma layering

Trauma layering refers to the idea that traumatic experiences can accumulate over time and form different layers. Here is a list of aspects that can be considered when looking at trauma layering:

1　Acute traumatic events: This includes single traumatic events that pose an immediate threat to life or physical integrity, such as a car accident or assault.
2　Complex traumatisation: This refers to repeated or prolonged traumatic experiences, such as child abuse, domestic violence or sexual abuse.
3　Developmental trauma: These are traumatic experiences that occur during a child's development and can affect confidence, security and self-esteem. These include neglect, separation from caregivers or emotional abuse.
4　Intergenerational trauma: This refers to traumatic experiences that can be passed on from one generation to the next. For example, a Holocaust survivor can pass on their traumatic experiences to their children.
5　Cultural trauma: This refers to traumatic events that affect an entire community or culture, such as wars, genocides or natural disasters.
6　Collective trauma: These are traumatic experiences that affect a larger group of people, such as terrorist attacks or pandemics.
7　Hidden trauma: This refers to traumatic experiences that may not be consciously remembered or recognised but can still have an impact on psychological well-being. This includes, for example, early childhood trauma or traumatic events that have been repressed in the subconscious.
8　Comorbid disorders: Trauma layering can also be associated with other mental disorders, such as anxiety disorders, depression or addictions.
9　Resilience and resources: It is important to recognise that despite traumatic experiences, people can have resilience and resources that can help them cope with the effects of trauma and recover.
10　Treatment options: When considering trauma layering, it is important to consider appropriate treatment options, such as prenatal-based psychotherapy and trauma therapy, depth psychotherapy, art psychotherapy, body psychotherapy, EMDR (eye movement desensitisation and reprocessing) or other evidence-based therapeutic approaches.

It is important to note that trauma layering is a complex issue and can vary from person to person.

> If we want to begin to understand our lives and those of our clients, we must be open to the infinite diversity of our life expressions and be prepared to go back a long way to understand them and, as I said, we must not

jump to conclusions. Seemingly "illogical" behaviour, "illogical" reactions or affects can emerge at any time as re-productions and re-enactments of very old experiences and *need to* be understood.

The fundamental characteristics of earliest experience are

1 Always individual and extremely complex in its appearance
2 Always unconscious or preconscious, preverbal and presymbolic
3 It is not obvious, does not present itself directly, but is rather hidden and concealed, fragmentary, irritating, incomprehensible, it eludes direct memorisation and yet urges to be understood
4 It bears within it the contradiction of the two soul registers according to J. Wilheim (p.52), that of the healthy register, to which we have access, and that of the sick register, which is not memorisable, only repeatable in its destructive tendency.
5 It contains our individual earliest relationship experiences, both the good and the bad, which include the relationship experiences of our ancestors. This means that our earliest experiences go far back before conception and before the beginning of our individual lives.

(Albrecht 2020, p. 4 f)

Case vignette: In a cancer patient's psychotherapy, an aetiological connection emerged from the fact that the first child was aborted in the female line over three generations, but further children were carried to term. The origin of the systemic trauma story lay in a forced abortion of the client's mother by her mother on the kitchen table because the love relationship was not appropriate. However, the couple stayed together and later had two children, including the patient. She aborted her first child as well as her daughter and niece. The hidden pain of the violent abortion of a couple's first child, which was actually very much wanted and loved, was thus unconsciously repeated in the next two generations in a trauma-compensatory manner.

Significance of prenatal psychology for psychotherapy

- Because of its formative implicit memory storage, the earliest trauma often seems to shape basic patterns of progression for later traumatic events. As an early sensorimotor "matrix", it obviously colours later traumatic experiences with regard to their affective and perceptual peculiarities. As it is often dissociatively fused with subsequent traumas, its activation potential can be constantly present in therapy, regardless of whether it can be addressed or not.

- The body as a "leading symptom carrier" in the process of imaginative-analytically oriented psychotherapy with early and complex traumatised patients (Hochauf 2007).
- Traumatisation in the pre-symbolic age has a particularly formative effect on future structural development due to the immature brain structure of the child. They are stored to a large extent in implicit and subcortical memory structures or mainly in the right hemisphere. The resulting post-traumatic syndromes are characterised in particular by sensorimotor-affective reactivation and symptomatic body fixation. Later childhood traumas become fixed to these via the dissociated qualities of the first break-off point, and the early traumas act as a sensorimotor matrix.
- This results in a time-fused dissociatively linked trauma layering that balances the structure in a trauma-compensatory manner. As the shock quality in trauma creates a permanent dissociation of psychological defence regulation and physical emergency programmes, the ability to experience the successful struggle for survival is of great importance for processing any trauma, which is made possible by working through the trauma layering. Prenatal trauma exposure is the basis and starting point for individual trauma stratification (Hochauf 2007, 2021).

The "Integrative Art and Body Therapy" developed by Evertz is intended to illustrate once again the therapeutic possibilities of deep regressive work (Evertz 2022).

As the traumas and stresses suffered took place before the development of the neocortical system, they cannot usually be consciously remembered. However, impulses, behaviours, symptoms of illness, dreams, inner images, movement patterns, paintings, etc. all contain memories of the physical self. On these levels, what is still closed to everyday consciousness can become visible. The patient can therefore be encouraged to enter into settings that address and activate these pre-linguistic memories and levels of expression. This includes, for example, spontaneous painting, breathing, psychodrama, many body therapy methods, music therapy but also scenic productions such as family constellations or concern constellations (according to Bert Hellinger and Franz Ruppert) or theatre therapy.

However, it is absolutely significant that the feelings triggered always remain in therapeutic contact. This means that an adult part of the patient's psyche always remains accessible, while the child parts are in regression. All sensations, feelings, images, etc. offered by the patient are perceived carefully and in a differentiated way and processed against the background of the possible biographical context and the individual trauma layering. Instead of a birth experience or a prenatal experience, for example, a postnatal trauma can of course also show up, such as a dangerous fall from the nappy-changing table that was not communicated in the family system.

Patients can follow all movement impulses so that they can also move freely in the room and/or want to be kept in physical contact with a group. A great deal of human expression is therefore possible. The main thing is that the patient is at the centre, that it is all about their story, that everything happens voluntarily and that it is always about the greatest protection of the inner child that is showing itself. All this is only possible if the therapist has a great deal of psychotherapeutic experience. These are always open processes, which means that the setting can reveal exactly what is most urgent in the patient's psyche at the time.

These are just brief references to modern open therapy methods that can initiate sustainable healing processes, especially in groups. However, there are no one-off miracle cures, but everything should be secured in a comprehensive therapy concept and often means years of educational and cognitive work for the patient. Ultimately, depth-psychological therapy methods are not just about curing a symptom but about initiating a lifelong process of enlightenment and development towards more mature forms of personality.

Special prenatal topics in psychotherapy

Basic trust
Loneliness
Being able to love and be loved
Fear of the world
Traumatic prenatal pain
Traumatic birth
Vanishing twin syndrome

In deep regressive therapeutic processes, the following perceptions and connections from the first, second and third trimester can emerge:

Perceived or executed movement:	Probable origin:
Floating with the feeling of being moved	Oocyte, before or after fertilisation.
Fish-like swimming	Sperm
Impact on the forehead	Implantation
Heavy pressure	Blastocyst, shortly after implantation
Floating and still, or limbs in motion	Foetus, first or second trimester
Fixed pressure	Third trimester and birth
Impact on head and shoulders	Birth

(Continued)

Scripts, impressions, feelings:	State of the mother:
She knows that I am here	Peaceful, happiness
She wants to get rid of me (choking)	Abortion attempted or considered
I am trembling so much; pain in the umbilical cord.	Mother's anxiety
I hate the cord, want her to love me	Sick mother, bedridden for a long time
It is warm, bliss to be cared for	Love
My feet, etc. are cold. Nobody cares	Early labour, incubator
Sharp hunger, painful, "it" doesn't come in	Neurotic mother, severe vomiting
Peaceful, movement	Cycling
Stay, feed me, love me	Husband is not here
I don't want a cord that pierces me	Cold, tense, like her own mother
Looks like a sea creature	Placenta
I feel impaled	Umbilical cord (tense and hard)
That is comforting (finger on the string)	Husband affirms wife and child

(cf. House 1999, p. 448)

This is only a small selection of possible sensations and perceptions in prenatal psychotherapy (Figure 9.8).

The degree of reality of these perceptions and messages from patients is astounding. Many prenatal therapists confirm these experiences. The decisive factor is the positive, lasting improvement in current symptoms following these experiences.

Stanislav Grof has identified four perinatal matrices for the birth event, which repeatedly become visible and can be named in therapeutic processes.

- Basic perinatal matrix I

  - Primordial unity with the mother
    The predominant feeling is that of being in a womb. The feelings are experienced positively, including oceanic feelings, feelings of unity with God or nature. It is about the experience of the original symbiotic unity of the foetus with the maternal organism in intrauterine existence. However, Grof also writes that bad emotional situations can sometimes prevail and then determine this matrix. Causes can be stress of the mother, alcohol consumption or somatic reasons.

- Basic perinatal matrix II

  - Antagonism with the mother
    The defining factor here is the painful experience of the onset of labour, characterised by uterine contractions and the opening of the uterine orifice. Images of hell arise, feelings of endless suffering, of being trapped and senselessness. Squeezing the head or the feeling of being threatened and injured by monsters is experienced as threatening.

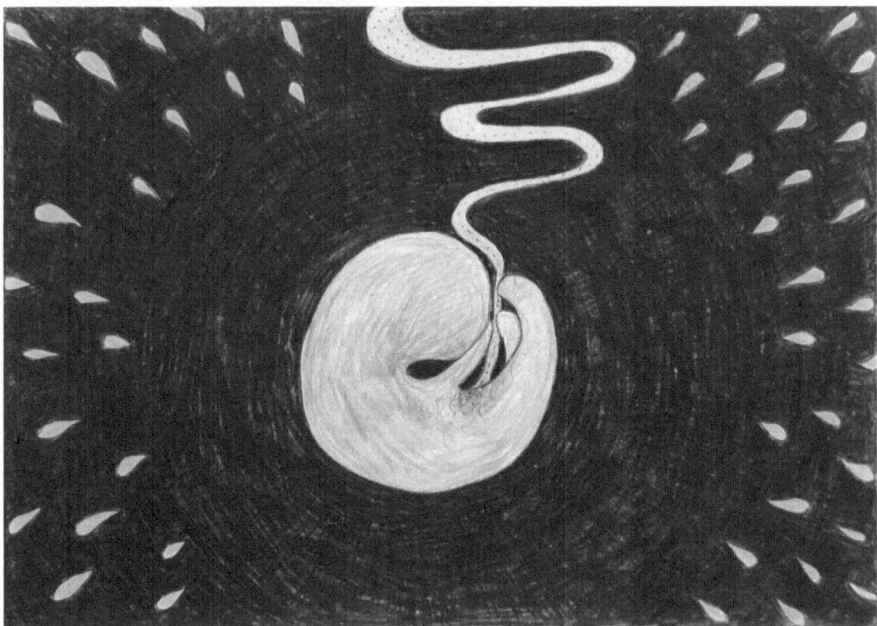

FIGURE 9.8   Illustration: Painting by an artist and art therapist whose mother was very young and very overwhelmed by the pregnancy.

PM II in particular is associated with fantasies of hell, which are characterised by never-ending physical torment, extreme pain, the idea of hot, confined spaces and the hopelessness of this situation.

- Basic perinatal matrix III
    - Synergy with the mother
      This matrix develops in the second clinical phase of biological birth; the uterine orifice is dilated, allowing the foetus to move gradually through the birth canal. Movement through the birth canal is central, linked to feelings of titanic struggle and massive mechanical pressure. Catastrophes, a mood of war, destruction, especially through the effects of water. Fantasies of ritual murders, sadomasochistic orgies and sacrifices dominate the scenarios. Excessive sexual arousal often arises during the activation of PM III, as well as scatological elements and the feeling of being hurt by fire.

- Basic perinatal matrix IV
    - Separation from the mother
      This matrix is created by being born and leaving the mother's body. This corresponds with the third clinical phase of labour, i.e. the delivery phase. The agonising birth struggle has come to an end. This separation

from the mother can be experienced as redemption, but also as total annihilation, as ego-death. At the end of the birth process, the "stepping out into the light of life" can be experienced.

• Corresponding psychopathological syndromes:
According to Grof, certain disorders can occur if the respective patterns of experience are insufficiently integrated. He assigns them to the basic perinatal matrices:

PM I: Schizophrenic psychoses (paranoid symptoms), feeling of mystical union; hypochondria; hysterical hallucinosis

PM II: Schizophrenic psychosis (perception of hellish ordeals), severely inhibited endogenous depression, irrational feelings of inferiority and guilt, hypochondria

PM III: Schizophrenic psychosis (sadomasochistic elements), agitated depression, sadomasochism, obsessive-compulsive neurosis, neurasthenia, organ neuroses

PM IV: Schizophrenic psychoses (death and rebirth experiences, delusional sense of mission) (cf. Grof 1975, p. 122ff)

All these levels are psychotherapeutically significant (Figure 9.9).

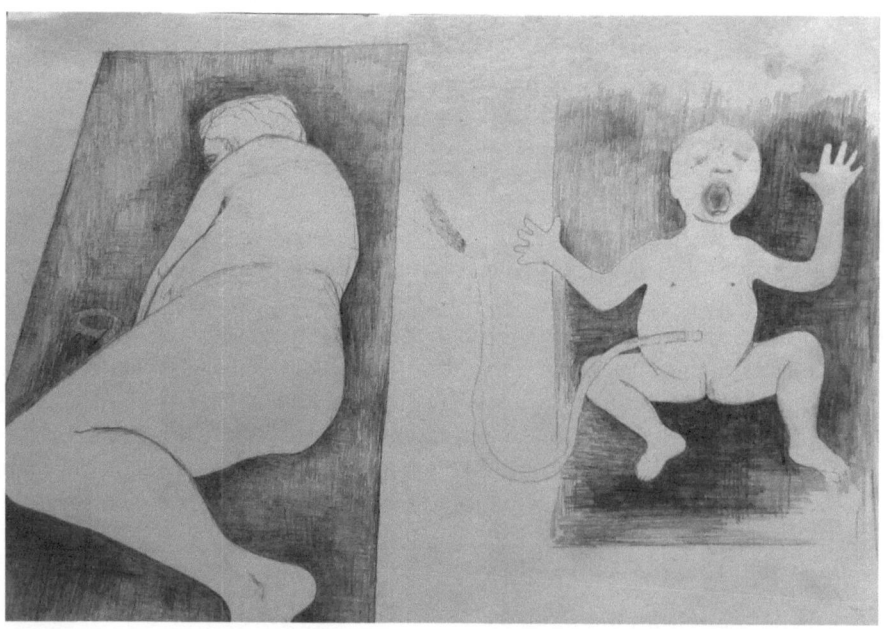

FIGURE 9.9 Drawing by an artist on the early distress of loneliness caused by her mother's departure.

In various psychotherapeutic settings, it has been observed time and again that the earliest pre-linguistic experiences before, during and after birth can appear in feelings and sensations. For example, it was possible to associate agonising sensations of compression on the head with a forceps birth, or feelings of constriction on the neck with an umbilical cord loop during birth. This was also possible for prenatal impairments, which could be reflected in later feelings of annihilation and suicide attempts. The discovery of these correlations was based on traumatic events, because they are reflected more clearly in later life. These observations formed a training ground for developing the perception of echoes of the earliest experiences in later life. For example, the mother's sensitivities and moods during pregnancy can influence how she feels later in life.

(Janus 2023, p. 13)

Wonderful paintings from art psychotherapies reflect the greatness of the earliest relationship qualities in the good, as well as in the threatening and in distress (Figures 9.10–9.14).

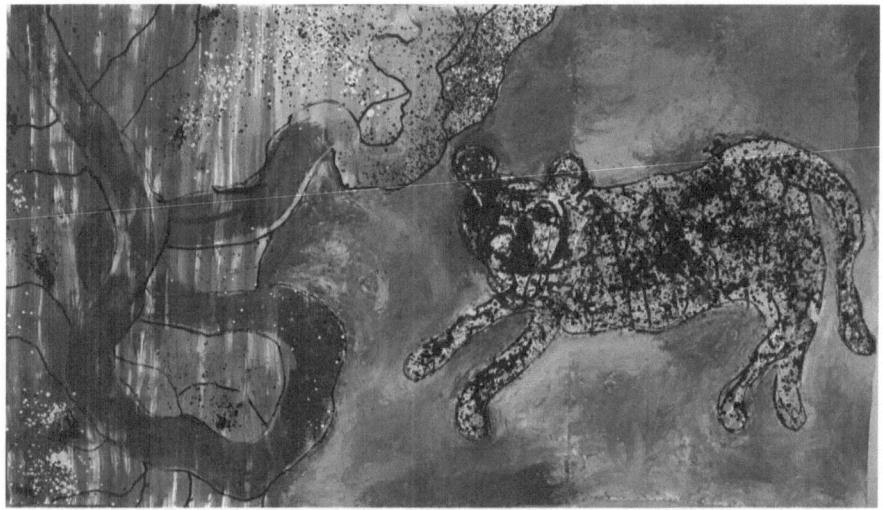

FIGURE 9.10 These four following paintings depict the confrontation of a 60-year-old artist and art therapist with the rejecting introjects of her mother, who became pregnant with her at the age of 18 and had a lot of other ideas for her life than becoming a mother at such an early age. The mother also remained ambivalent towards the child postnatally. The first picture with the predator shows her own determination and anger to approach the umbilical cord feelings of her prenatal period.

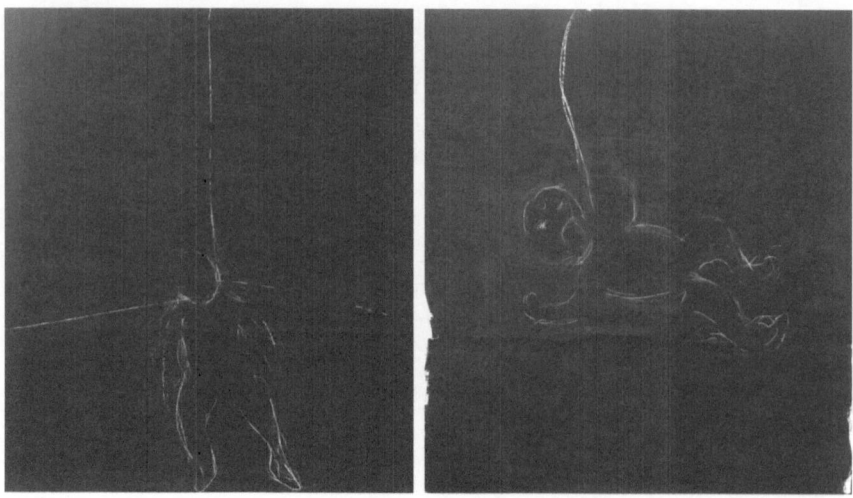

FIGURE 9.11A Two other large-format pictures show the distress of the child on the threshold of fears of annihilation, including the fear of being strangled by the umbilical cord.

FIGURE 9.11B Two other large-format pictures show the distress of the child on the threshold of fears of annihilation, including the fear of being strangled by the umbilical cord.

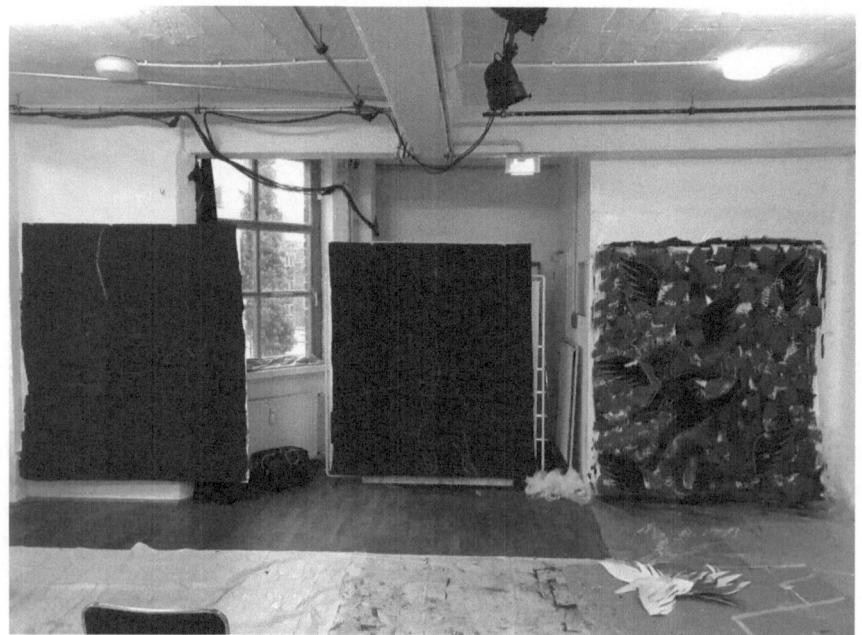

FIGURE 9.12 This picture shows the art psychotherapy setting with three pictures.

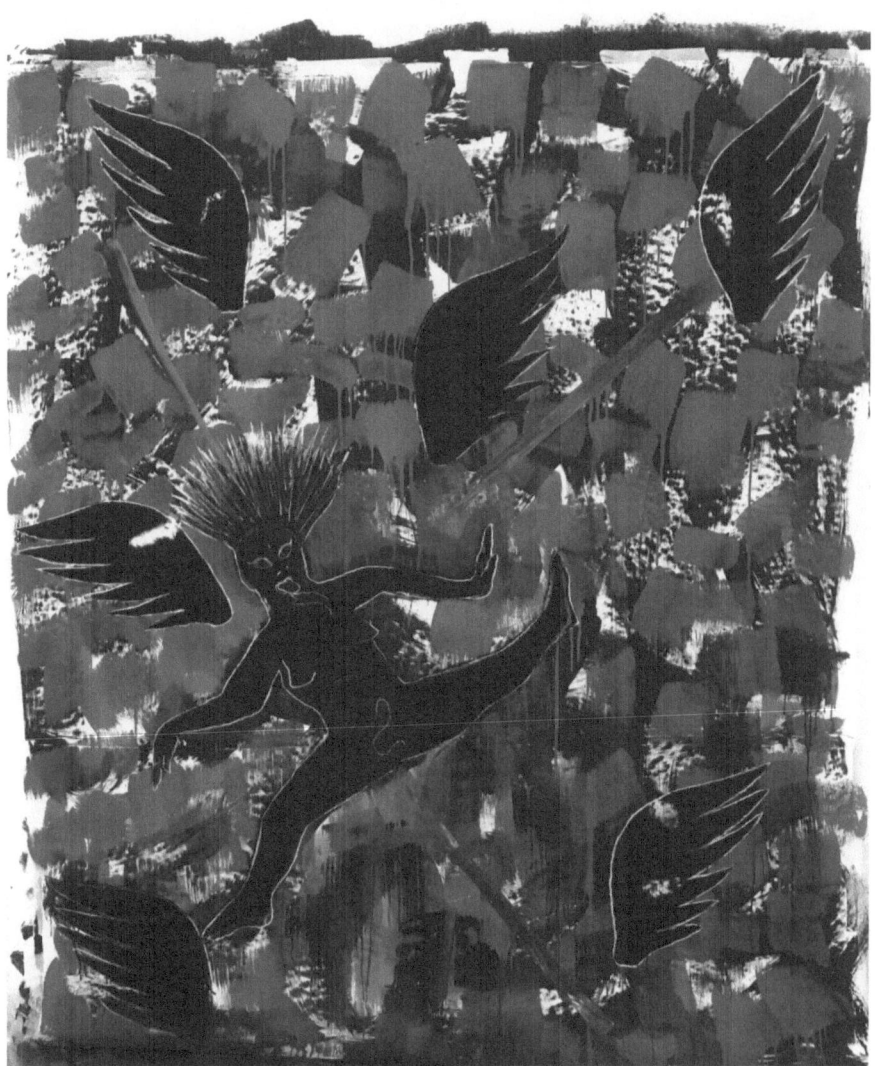

FIGURE 9.13   The fourth picture shows the tension, the inner distress: as if electrified, energised, in the mother's ambivalence to decide for or against the child. This series of pictures triggered many new possibilities and healing potentials. Finally, everything that had always caused so much inner fear and anxiety could be looked at and expressed.

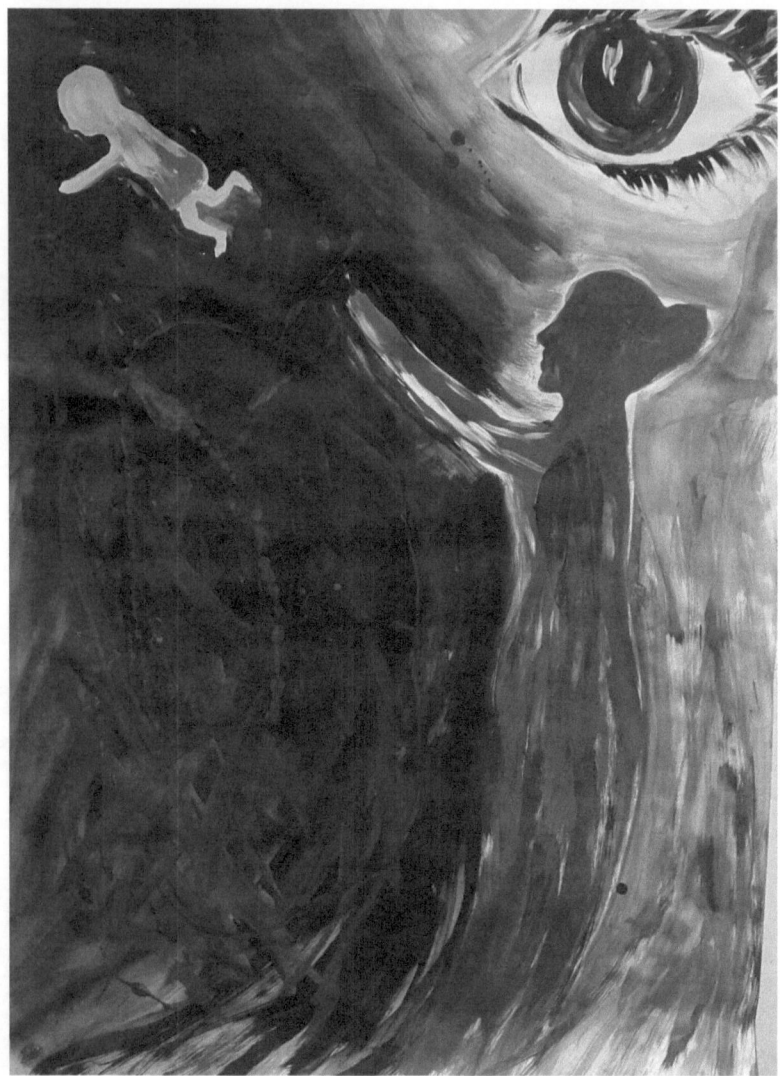

FIGURE 9.14 Children have to be sacrificed when the mother cannot be a mother because of her history. Painting of a client who suffered from her mother's abortion fantasies.

Summary

Prenatal-based psychotherapy and psychotraumatology open up a new understanding of many physical and mental illnesses that we have previously tried to summarise in general nosology in unclear aetiologies.

A fundamental expansion of previous psychotherapy is both the expansion of therapeutic knowledge and the expansion of therapeutic means. Body-psychotherapeutic methods, psychodramatic and music-therapeutic methods, art-psychotherapeutic methods and depth-psychology-based forms of psychotherapy can all complement each other to form a prenatal-based psychotherapy.

Literature

Albrecht G (2020) Frühestes Erleben in seiner Präsenz, lecture 2020 at the St. Georg conference and guest house, Cologne, unpublished.

Emerson W (2021) "Psychotherapy with infants and children". In: Evertz K et al. (eds.) *Handbook for prenatal psychology – Integrating research and practice.* Springer Nature, Heidelberg, New York, 543–558.

Evertz K (2020) "The inner child or the "inner child"? Confusion during pregnancy and its lifelong consequences". In: Gouni O et al. (eds.) *Change – Birthing & parenting at times of crisis.* Cosmoanelixis, Athens, 2021, 293–334.

Evertz K (2022) "Sensing the world anew – The transgenerational-systemic and prenatal method-integrative psychotherapy – Integrative art and body therapy". In: Klippel-Heidekrüger M, Janus L (eds.) *Diverse approaches to pre-linguistic and natal experience.* Mattes, Heidelberg, 271–292.

Evertz K, Janus L, Linder R (2021) *Handbook of prenatal and perinatal psychology.* Springer Nature, Cham, New York.

Grof Stanislav (1975) *Topography of the unconscious: LSD in the service of depth psychological research.* Klett-Cotta, Stuttgart.

Hermer M, Röhrle B (2008) *Handbuch der therapeutischen Beziehung.* dgvt-Verlag, Tübingen.

Hirsch M (2004) *Psychoanalytische Traumatologie – Das Trauma in der Familie.* Schattauer, Stuttgart.

Hochauf R (2007) *Early trauma and structural deficit.* Asanger, Kröning.

Hochauf R (2021) "Analytical psychotherapy and the access to early trauma". In: Evertz K, Janus L, Linder R (eds.) *Handbook of prenatal and perinatal psychology.* Springer Nature, Cham, New York, 419–448.

Hochauf R (2023) Lecture announcement. Unpublished.

House S (1999) "Primal integration therapy -School of Lake". In: *International Journal of Prenatal and Perinatal Psychology and Medicine* 11(4): 437–457.

Janus L (ed.) (2013) *The prenatal dimension in psychotherapy.* Mattes, Heidelberg.

Janus L (2023) *The psychological dimension of pregnancy and birth.* Mattes, Heidelberg.

Lambert MJ, Barley DE (2001) "Research summary on the therapeutic relationship and psychotherapy outcome". In: *Psychotherapy: Theory, Research, Practice, Training* 38(4): 357–361. https://doi.org/10.1037/0033-3204.38.4.357

Linder R (2021) "Love, pregnancy, conflict and solution: on the way to an understanding of conflicted pregnancy". In: Evertz K, Janus L, Linder R (eds.) *Handbook of Prenatal and Perinatal Psychology*, Springer Nature, Cham, 337–346.

Linderkamp O (2014) "Brain development and early support". In: Evertz K, et al. (eds.) *Textbook of prenatal psychology.* Mattes, Heidelberg, 19–33.

Ott M, Singer M, Bliem HR, Schubert C (2021) "Prenatal psychoneuroimmunology". In: Evertz K, Janus L, Linder R (eds.) *Handbook of prenatal and perinatal psychology*. Springer, New York, S. 115–158.

Roth G (2014) Feeling, thinking, acting. Suhrkamp, Frankfurt.

Terry K (2014) " Pre- and perinatal baby therapy". In: Evertz K, Janus L, Linder R (eds.) *Textbook of prenatal psychology*. Mattes, Heidelberg, 425–436.

Verdult R (2014) "Pränatale Bindungsentwicklung – auf dem Weg zu einer pränatalen Entwicklungspsychologie". In: Evertz K, Janus L, Linder R (eds.) *Lehrbuch der Pränatalen Psychologie*. Mattes, Heidelberg, 205–231.

10

CONCLUSION

Prenatal psychology (PP) is a scientific discipline that initially encompasses the following transdisciplinary levels:

1 Medical–psychological–therapeutic meaning
2 Cultural-psychological, philosophical and anthropological significance

Through PP, we not only gain an expanded nosological understanding but also an expanded anthropological and philosophical understanding of the prenatal existence of the human being and thus a new view of human existence in general. Today, thanks to prenatal medicine and psychology, we can locate the beginning of the aetiology of almost all diseases in the prenatal phase of life. This gives us a fundamentally expanded level of medical and psychological interventions so that we can speak of a paradigm shift.

In terms of cultural psychology, PP can initiate a second enlightenment by revealing many previously unrecognised projections in human culture and science. The trauma-generated projections from prenatal times can be recognised, and thus, many dissociative patterns in human thought and action can be understood and resolved.

The PP is therefore one of the important keys to the future emancipation of global humanity towards a peaceful world society.

Medical–psychological–therapeutic meaning

In psychotherapy, PP enables us for the first time to clearly differentiate and treat transgenerational, pre- and perinatal and postnatal traumatisation and stress in people's biographies.

DOI: 10.4324/9781003480242-10

As a result, the medical aetiologies or aetiological hypotheses of somatic and mental illnesses and disorders, some of which were previously inadequate, can now be supplemented by psychosomatic aetiologies and diagnoses and treatment options that were not possible just a few years ago. Today, we can fundamentally expand and complement the biomedical model of illness towards a bio-psycho-social medicine and psychology that does not work competitively or mutually exclusive but can offer integrative, comprehensive diagnoses and therapies (Engel 1977; Janus 2024; Evertz 2021, 2022).

The paradigm shift lies particularly in the fact that we not only fill the aetiological gap between the biological-genetic explanations and the explanations based solely on postnatal risk factors but also decisively expand it through prenatal epigenetics and prenatal programming and prenatal psychology. In fact, today we have to locate the centre of gravity and beginning of most vulnerabilities, the starting point of allostatic burden and thus most aetiologies in pregnancy. The disposition to the vast majority of later illnesses lies in the prenatal phase of life (see Chapter 3).

In future, we will have to take greater account of biological, psychological and social factors in their complex interactions in the development and maintenance of diseases even during pregnancy. The traditional genetic and postnatal, purely biomedically orientated understanding of disease with its dichotomous view is no longer sufficient for researching, diagnosing and treating chronic diseases in particular: Chronic diseases cannot be reduced to a somatogenic or psychogenic core or a mere addition of somatic and psychological factors.

The body self of every human being begins with the zygote and is already determined by the experiences of the parents and previous generations but is then permanently exposed to interactions and exchange processes in the biotope of the maternal environment. The child creates itself from these complex, dynamic interactions. The prenatal development phase is the fundamental condition of life as a whole.

A holistic understanding of our existence can fundamentally expand our nosology and help avoid malpractice.

Significant reductions in pregnancy and birth complications can be achieved decisively by integrating the attachment and relationship psychology findings of PP, especially attachment analysis (Goertz-Schroth et al. 2023). More social empathy for the beginning of life saves huge costs in the health sector for later postnatal illnesses and disorders of all kinds.

The findings of PP are indispensable for all doctors and therapists who work in the context of pregnancy and birth, with infants, children, adolescents, adults and families, for active researchers, basic and translational scientists and clinicians in the fields of human genetics, genomics, reproductive medicine, gynaecology, obstetrics, andrology, embryology, endocrinology, bioinformatics, prenatal testing, psychology, psychiatry and genetic testing, as well as for genetic counsellors and bioethicists.

Population-political, cultural-psychological, philosophical and anthropological significance

Friedrich Nietzsche "Man is not only an individual, but the living whole-organic in a certain line".

(Estate 1886/1887, KSA 12, 7[2])

We must assume that the nature-made disasters and the man-made disasters of human history have left and continue to leave strong dissociative aspects in the cultural-historical models that we have made of the world over the last 10,000 years. This applies to mythological, religious, artistic and philosophical models as well as to scientific models of the world. However, the Enlightenment has already created a less projectively burdened level through the foundation of science, which is already less dissociatively burdened than the previous models of explaining the world. Nevertheless, we can speak of a post-traumatic stress disorder of humanity that still has a negative and sabotaging effect in all political, cultural and scientific contexts.

PP as the Second Enlightenment can today further detach our view of the world from trauma-generated projections than before, as these can only be seen through and understood by PP. The strange splits and rescue illusions, e.g. in the categories "consciousness" and "soul" and the body-mind-spirit models or the matter-spirit opposition, historically understandable, reveal themselves as dissociative. Matter and spirit are ontologically one, it is more a question of complexity of a single ontological basis, and our previous cultural division models turn out to be collective inner-psychic compromises and trauma-compensatory measures of previous human fear and distress, if they are not consciously used for heuristic purposes. The concept of an "ontological consciousness" can overcome the old divisions in an integrative way and describe the potential of the human being to be able to grasp all physical, mental and spiritual experiences from the first cell onwards, including the transgenerational sums of information, unconsciously/consciously and also tend to be able to sense, feel and think. (This was called transmigration of souls, karma, etc. in earlier religious references.)

Questions about the seat of consciousness, the soul or the spirit in the brain reveal a certain average immaturity of introspection and interoceptive perception. For humans, sensations are always whole-bodied and so all the foundations of our feeling and thinking are always whole-bodied, but we then become entangled in dissociative models of wholeness and argue about biology or psychology, although they are only different approaches to one and the same reason: experiential realities of the body self.

Post-materialist science assumes that there is a connection between the biomolecular processes of the brain and the basic structure of the universe (precisely because the brain emerged from the evolutionary process).

Quantum coherence has been demonstrated in plant photosynthesis, navigation in the bird brain and the human sense of smell.

(Verny 2021, p. 157)

The fact that the destructive aggression and auto-aggression of mankind is not an anthropological constant, but a collective disorder at the deepest affective level, an average post-traumatic stress of human populations, explains the excesses and extreme crimes and the lust for destruction, as we have been able to observe in the therapeutic culture over the last 100 years in millions of individual psychological enlightenment processes in therapies. The staging of wars is a psychotic phenomenon and cannot be explained without the level of prenatal and perinatal trauma, i.e. the deepest affects.

Humanity's blindness to the true origin of destruction (Janus 2024) is revealed more deeply by the PP. The world would have room for a peaceful life for all people and could easily feed 10 billion people, but instead, there is still too much destructiveness. Where does this actually come from?

The future of global society will largely depend on how the new generations feel and learn from the outset that the world can be a good place that can be shaped and developed peacefully. Traumatic experiences in the prenatal phase generally lead to difficult life stagings, including significantly increased dispositions to illness, but also an increased likelihood of destructive social and political stagings of all kinds. The paranoid is always anti-familial and antisocial!

The task of making the first intrauterine months of life and birth as safe as possible is therefore one of the most essential requirements of a modern health policy and a future democratically organised global society.

In his outline of the world bonding theory (Evertz 2013), Evertz traced the four greatest current threats to humanity back to four different prenatal traumatisations of the average world population:

1 Ecological danger – parasitic paradigm
2 Religious fundamentalism – rescue illusion paradigm
3 Economic-political power struggles – abortive paradigm
4 Ideological and ideological constraints – paradigm of constraints

It is precisely through PP that we learn that our relationship to the world is originally and essentially characterised by the quality of the relationship between father, mother and child. That we have a feeling of coherence, a feeling of continuity, of a coherent reality of experience! A securely bonded child from a securely bonded and loving couple perceives the world and reality in a much more connected and coherent way than a child from a dysfunctional couple relationship, who has to learn to perceive the world in a much more fragmented and fearful way! Of course, we also find these qualities of continuity and fragmentation in all kinds of scientific models and their interpretations, even with originally identical data!

This means that PP is not only an extension of developmental psychology as part of psychology or psychological anthropology but also brings about a new understanding of a new scientific approach that can take a much more open and related view of the relationship between man and the world.

It is about developing mature parental competence for global processes. Humanity is increasingly assuming parental responsibility for itself and the world (Grille 2005). Since the declaration of universal human rights in 1949, the founding of the UN, the establishment of an International Court of Justice, the improvement of diplomatic and communicative networks worldwide, there are clearly more empathic, i.e. more mature, more adult levels of responsibility (Rifkin 2010). Nevertheless, humanity's traumatic history still gives rise to an abundance of mistrust and paranoia, which hinder cooperation and development and promote atavism.

Every love relationship, every family is, so to speak, a new evolutionary attempt to find out how human coexistence can succeed better and better. However, the possibility of entering into a relationship with a partner, of living real "love relationships", which has become much more complex and free since the Enlightenment, also means that the individual man and woman have a greater responsibility to constructively see through and dissolve the various projections, fantasies and idealisations, as well as the attachment qualities learned in the family, in the new relationship and to be able to develop them into more mature levels of attachment. This also applies to same-sex relationships.

Basic family conditions are: Empathy and mutual responsibility, trust and working on individual and joint development, being able to resolve emotional deficiencies, not in the sense of abundance at the expense of other family members, but of balance and sustainability. Everyone must have their place in the system, and everyone needs to be recognised and appreciated.

A good indication of family success is the ability of a family to allow itself feelings, both in happiness and in constructive conflict, without abortion levels being involved. This means that even the most violent anger about behaviour in the family can be dealt with without abandonment or being abandoned, exclusion or even injury and violence leading to new traumatisation. The old burdens of the family history in the transgenerational flow must be recognised as such, identified as introjects and healed so that they can no longer sabotage or even make impossible a family development towards self-responsibility, autonomy, justice, trust and love.

According to WHO estimates, 41% of pregnancies worldwide are unintended (WHO 2022). A recent study (BZgA 2016) from Germany found that around a third (33.7%) of pregnancies were unintended (unwanted/ambiguous/wanted, but later). Almost 18% of these pregnancies were explicitly unintended, but more than half of them (57%) were carried to term (Pro Familia 2016).

This data provides important information about the "self-inflicted immaturity" (Kant) of human society and the political necessity of forcing scientific education and parallel psychosocial support for pregnant couples worldwide in order to further reduce future man-made disasters on the way to a predominantly peaceful and just world society of the future. All the positive figures, e.g. the fact that around 500,000 babies no longer die perinatally every year as a result of the improved global birth culture, indicate that the earlier investments are made in good conditions for human development, the greater the return will be.

If we consider the dramatic collapse in global fertility described in a study recently published in the medical journal *The Lancet*, it becomes clear that human life has reached a point where there are strong inhibitions to further reproduction. According to the study, global fertility more than halved between 1950 and 2021. (GBD 2021)

Is this due to a responsible population policy in view of the threat of overpopulation or a depressive turn of events?

Everyone benefits when we invest in, promote and support the early development of the world's greatest natural resource – people.

PP impressively traces contemporary efforts for more empathy, more healing, more enlightenment, more truthfulness back to the deeper real causes of individual and collective pathologies and offers a broad spectrum of concrete practical possibilities for healing, emancipation and improving living conditions. The infinite helplessness, delicacy, vulnerability of all our beginnings in life, of which we are still so afraid, practise denial and therefore as a human society still stage so much self-harm, can be recognised more clearly in the traumatic endangerment.

These traumatic and frightening aspects block the inner contact to our prenatal self and to our original vitality and creativity, which we have historically always localised as a higher world outside.

Through the confrontation with the earliest traumatic aspects that is now possible, this inner original image can become accessible again as our own and become the source of our strength and humanity in later life.

This is also the core of future emancipatory-democratic achievements: to become individually and collectively capable of working on the early and earliest childhood pain instead of having to project and act it out. And consequently, to decisively advance multidisciplinary prophylaxis in the sense of a general, comprehensive "immunology".

Through PP, humanity can therefore learn to take a more loving view of itself. We can learn that bonding and relationship processes can be

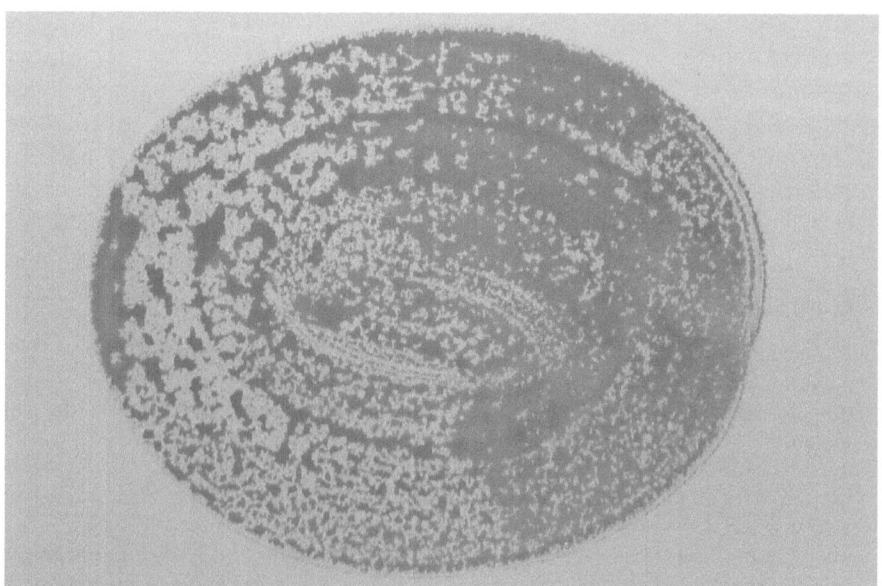

FIGURE 10.1   Evertz K. Farbhandlung 21.7.21, 50 × 60 cm, acrylic, HDF.

developed further, that love can be understood and developed more comprehensively and responsibly, that love between generations can be appreciated more obviously, that the interconnectedness of all life can ultimately be protected more and that an empathic civilisation becomes increasingly possible.

More peaceful societies are possible. Destructive aggression is not an anthropological constant. Humanity's post-traumatic stress disorders from past catastrophes, such as high infant mortality rates, wars, hunger and disease, merciless distribution struggles, idealisations of destructiveness and paranoia, political compulsions of fear can be understood more and more in their origins and then no longer need to be restaged (Figure 10.1) (DeMause 1982, 2000).

1 PP is the foundation of all developmental psychology and attachment psychology and should therefore also be the developmental psychological foundation of all psychotherapeutic models.
2 The aetiology of almost all diseases in childhood, adolescence and adulthood can now be traced back to the genetics and epigenetics of pregnancy (DOHAD).
3 All human behavioural patterns and bonding abilities have their starting point in the prenatal phase of life: being-in-the-mother is the decisive matrix for being-in-the-world.

4 Global peace society – real peace work: by recognising and resolving the earliest traumas and becoming aware of the earliest fears, a peaceful society can be prepared and strengthened. The more conscious parenthood becomes possible, the more the global society can assume real parental responsibility for itself and the world.
5 In terms of cultural psychology, PP provides a more comprehensive understanding of the power of the arts and the invention of religions (Evertz 2021b).

Literature

DeMause L (1982) *Foundations of psychohistory*. Creative Books, New York.
DeMause L (2000) *Was ist Psychohistorie?* Psychosozial, Gießen.
Engel GL (1977) "The need for a new model: A challenge for biomedicine". In: *Science* 196: 129–137.
Evertz K (2013) "Aspekte einer Weltbindungstheorie". In: Janus L (ed.) *Die Psychologie der Mentalitätsentwicklung – vom archaischen Bewusstsein zum modernen Bewusstsein*. LIT Verlag, Münster, 173–188.
Evertz K (2021) "Prenatal Psychology holdsthe key: Thoughts about the cultural Meaning of Prenatal Psychology". In: Evertz K, Janus L, Linder R (eds.) *Handbook of prenatal and perinatal psychology*. Springer Nature, Cham, New York, 783–798.
Evertz K (2022) "Die Welt neu spüren – Die transgenerational-systemisch und pränatal fundierte methodenintegrative Psychotherapie – Integrative Kunst- und Körpertherapie". In: Klippel-Heidekrüger M, Janus L (eds.) *Vielfältige Zugänge zum vorsprachlichen und geburtlichen Erleben*. Mattes Verlag, Heidelberg, 271–292.
Evertz K, Janus L, Linder R (2021) *Handbook of prenatal and perinatal psychology*. Springer Nature, Cham, New York.
GBD 2021 Fertility and Forecasting Collaborators. Global Fertility in 204 Countries and Territories, 1950–2021, With Forecasts to 2100: A Comprehensive Demographic Analysis for the Global Burden of Disease Study 2021. *The Lancet* 2024; 403(10440): 2057-2099. DOI: https://doi.org/10.1016/S0140-6736(24)00550-6.
Goertz-Schroth A, Schroth G, Phillips R (2023) "Prenatal Bonding (BA) as a breakthrough in improving pregnancy, birth, and postpartum outcomes". In: *Journal for Prenatal and Perinatal Psychology and Health* 37(1), 1–21.
Grille R (2005) *Parenting for a peaceful world*. Vox Cordis Press, Alexandria.
Janus L (2023) *The psychological dimension of pregnancy and birth*. Mattes, Heidelberg.
Janus L (2024) *The enduring effects of prenatal experiences – Echoes from the womb*. Newcastle, Cambridge Scholars Publishing.
Pro Familia: BZgA Federal Centre for Health Education (ed.) (2016) *frauen leben 3. Familienplanung im Lebenslauf von Frauen. Focus on unwanted pregnancies*. A study commissioned by the BZgA by Cornelia Helfferich, Heike Klindworth, Yvonne Heine, Ines Wlosnewski. Cologne: BZgA. Online at: publikationen. sexualaufklae rung.de/index.php?docid=4043 (accessed: 5.2.18).
Rifkin J (2010) *The empathic civilisation*. Campus, Frankfurt.
Verny T (2021) *The embodied mind. Understanding the mysteries of cellular memory, consciousness and our bodies*. Pegasus Books, New York, London.
WHO (2022) https://www.who.int/news/item/24-03-2022-first-ever-country-level-estimates-of-unintended-pregnancy-and-abortion

INDEX

Note: **Bold** page numbers refer to tables and *italic* page numbers refer to figures.